Essential Neuroanatomy

Vijay Yanamadala

Essential Neuroanatomy

A Pocket Guide for Medical Students and Residents

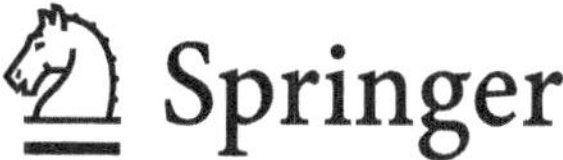

Vijay Yanamadala
Neurosurgery
Hartford Healthcare and Quinnipiac University
Westport, CT, USA

ISBN 978-3-032-26876-1 ISBN 978-3-032-26877-8 (eBook)
https://doi.org/10.1007/978-3-032-26877-8

This Springer imprint is published by the registered company Springer Nature Switzerland AG
The registered company address is: Gewerbestrasse 11, 6330 Cham, Switzerland

To my grandparents, who inspired me to become a surgeon—and who taught me that knowledge finds its highest purpose when it heals.

Preface

The purpose of this book is to efficiently provide students with the essentials of neuroanatomy that every medical student, neuroscience student, and clinician in training should know. Having served as a neurosurgery resident, fellow, and attending at institutions where neuroanatomy is taught in the context of real operative and clinical decisions, I came to appreciate that no current text strikes the right balance between structural detail and functional relevance. With an ever-expanding body of neuroscience knowledge and ever-shrinking curricular time, my goal in writing this book has been to give you everything you need to know—and nothing more.

Neuroanatomy has a reputation that precedes it: the subject that humbles even the most confident students. The brain and spinal cord are, by any measure, the most complex structures in the known universe, and the temptation when studying them is to either give up in the face of their complexity or to descend into an endless catalog of nuclei, tracts, and eponymous syndromes that seems to have no bottom. Neither approach serves you well. What I have tried to do in this book is offer a third path—one grounded in the principle that structure only becomes meaningful when understood in the context of function, and that function only becomes clinically useful when it can be localized.

In using this book, your goal should be twofold: (1) to understand which structural lesions produce which clinical syndromes, and (2) to understand which functional systems are most vulnerable to disease and why. Every tract, every nucleus, every vascular territory described in these pages should be read through that lens. When you encounter the corticospinal tract, ask not merely where it runs, but what happens when it is compressed by a herniated disc, damaged by a stroke in the internal capsule, or demyelinated in multiple sclerosis. When you encounter the limbic system, ask not merely which structures comprise it, but how its disruption manifests in memory, mood, and behavior. Neuroanatomy approached this way stops being an exercise in memorization and becomes instead a language—one that lets you read a patient's examination and hear exactly where the nervous system is speaking from.

The importance of neuroanatomy within medicine is growing, not diminishing. Advances in neuroimaging now allow us to visualize structural pathology at submillimeter resolution in real time. Intraoperative neuromonitoring demands that surgeons and anesthesiologists understand functional anatomy well enough to interpret evoked potential changes on the fly. Deep brain stimulation, spinal cord stimulation, focused ultrasound, and the emerging field of closed-loop neuromodulation all require a precision of anatomical knowledge that was once the exclusive domain of subspecialists. Understanding neuroanatomy is no longer optional for anyone who cares for patients with diseases of the nervous system—which is to say, nearly everyone in medicine.

Much of the material in this book grew out of notes I compiled over years of teaching medical students, residents, and fellows—first informally, at the bedside and in the operating room, and later more systematically as I developed a clinical and academic practice centered on the spine and complex neurosurgical reconstruction. Like the biochemistry textbook that preceded it, this text began as a set of distilled, high-yield materials that learners found more useful than any single comprehensive reference. Colleagues and students encouraged me over many years to formalize those materials into a book that others could benefit from. It is my sincere hope that I have done justice to that encouragement.

A number of people made this book possible. My residents and medical students across many years asked the questions that sharpened my thinking and forced me to articulate things I had previously only intuited. My mentors in neurosurgery modeled the kind of anatomical precision that I have tried to transmit here. My parents instilled in me the belief that knowledge, freely shared, is knowledge multiplied. My wife Vidya—herself a physician who understands better than anyone the demands of a life in academic medicine—has supported this project with a patience and generosity I can never fully repay, along with the steadfast encouragement of my father-in-law and mother-in-law, without which this final version could never have come together. And my children, Rishi and Meera, who inspire me every single day to be worthy of the curiosity they bring to the world—this book is, in no small part, for them. Above all, I am grateful to each patient who has entrusted their care to me. To allow another person to operate on your brain or spine is an act of profound trust, and it is that trust—more than anything else—that has made me a better student of anatomy than any textbook ever could.

With all my best,

Westport, CT, USA Vijay Yanamadala

Contents

1 **The Spinal Cord** 1

2 **The Brainstem** 27

3 **The Cranial Nerves** 61

4 **The Cerebellum** 79

5 **The Diencephalon** 103

6 **The Basal Ganglia** 123

7 **The Cerebral Cortex** 139

8 **The Ventricular System and Hydrocephalus** 189

9 **Blood Supply of the Central Nervous System** 203

10 **Neurodevelopment** 237

Index 261

About the Author

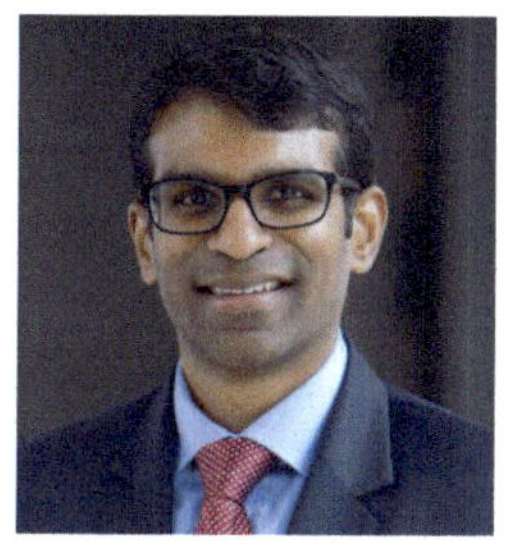

Vijay Yanamadala, MD, MBA, FAANS, FCNS, is a board-certified neurosurgeon who specializes in complex and revision spine surgery. He completed his undergraduate studies at Harvard University, where he studied biochemistry, and completed a master's degree in organic chemistry at Harvard University, prior to earning his MD at Harvard Medical School. He earned his MBA at Harvard Business School. He completed his residency in neurological surgery at Massachusetts General Hospital, in addition to a fellowship in orthopedic spine surgery at Massachusetts General Hospital and a fellowship in complex spine surgery and spinal deformity at Virginia Mason Medical Center.

He currently serves as Vice Chairman of Neurosurgery and System Medical Director of Quality, Innovation & Research at the Ayer Neuroscience Institute, Hartford HealthCare, the largest healthcare system in the state of Connecticut. He is Associate Professor of Neurosurgery at the Quinnipiac University Frank H. Netter School of Medicine. He has extensive teaching experience across medical biochemistry, neuroanatomy, and clinical neuroscience.

In his clinical practice, he treats complex spinal disorders, including scoliosis, spinal deformity, spine trauma, and spinal vascular disease, with a particular focus on revision surgery and the avoidance of unnecessary procedures. He is a pioneering surgeon who was among the first in Connecticut to offer awake spinal fusion surgery and was the second surgeon in the world to offer patient-specific spine fusion surgery. He has performed international spine surgery missions in Kenya, India, Mongolia, and Sri Lanka. He has published over 95 peer-reviewed scientific papers, authored two medical textbooks, and received numerous awards for safe and effective treatment of complex spinal conditions.

He previously served as Chief Medical Officer of Sword Health. He is a 2008 Paul & Daisy Soros Fellow, certified by the Safety in Spine Surgery Project (S3P), and is a Fellow of the American Association of Neurological Surgeons and the Congress of Neurological Surgeons, and a member of the North American Spine Society and the Scoliosis Research Society.

The Spinal Cord 1

Introduction

The spinal cord is a long, cylindrical structure extending from the medulla oblongata at the base of the brain to the lumbar vertebrae in the lower back. As a crucial component of the central nervous system (CNS), it serves as the primary pathway for transmitting sensory and motor information between the brain and the rest of the body. A useful clinical analogy describes the spinal cord as the "telephone cord" connecting our brain with our body, facilitating bidirectional communication essential for voluntary movement, sensation, and autonomic regulation.

Beyond its role in signal transmission, the spinal cord independently processes and coordinates reflexes and autonomic functions, demonstrating considerable integrative capacity. Encased within the protective vertebral column, the spinal cord's internal architecture comprises gray matter (neuronal cell bodies and synapses), white matter (myelinated axon tracts), and a central canal containing cerebrospinal fluid. Understanding this organization is fundamental to comprehending both normal neurological function and the pathophysiology of spinal cord disorders.

V. Yanamadala, *Essential Neuroanatomy*,
https://doi.org/10.1007/978-3-032-26877-8_1

Gross Anatomy of the Spinal Cord

Location and Extent

In adults, the spinal cord measures approximately 45 cm (18 inches) in length, extending from the medulla oblongata at the base of the brainstem to the L1-L2 vertebral level (first or second lumbar vertebra). This discrepancy between spinal cord length and vertebral column length results from differential growth rates during development and has important clinical implications for procedures such as lumbar puncture.

Spinal cord segments:

- *Cervical region*: Uppermost part, consisting of eight cervical segments (C1-C8), controlling neck, diaphragm, and upper limb function.
- *Thoracic region*: Middle portion, consisting of 12 thoracic segments (T1-T12), innervating the trunk and containing sympathetic neurons.
- *Lumbar region*: Lower part, consisting of five lumbar segments (L1-L5), providing innervation to the lower trunk and portions of the lower limbs.
- *Sacral region*: Consisting of five sacral segments (S1-S5), controlling the lower limb, pelvic floor, and bowel/bladder function.
- *Coccygeal region*: Terminal part with one coccygeal segment (Co1), providing limited sensory innervation to the coccygeal region.

Regional Anatomy and Variations

The cross-sectional appearance of the spinal cord varies significantly at different levels, reflecting the functional demands of each region. These variations in the relative amounts of gray and white matter, as well as the presence of specialized nuclei, are clinically significant for localization of spinal pathology.

- *Upper cervical cord*: Characterized by abundant white matter and relatively sparse gray matter; contains the spinal accessory nucleus (controlling trapezius and sternocleidomastoid muscles) and phrenic nucleus (C3-C5, innervating the diaphragm).
- *Lower cervical cord*: Features substantial white matter with prominent anterior horn enlargements corresponding to the motor neuron pools innervating the upper limbs; forms the cervical enlargement. Figure 1.1 depicts a cross section of the cervical spinal cord at the level of C7.
- *Thoracic region*: Lacks the fasciculus cuneatus (present only above T6); contains relatively small amounts of gray matter;

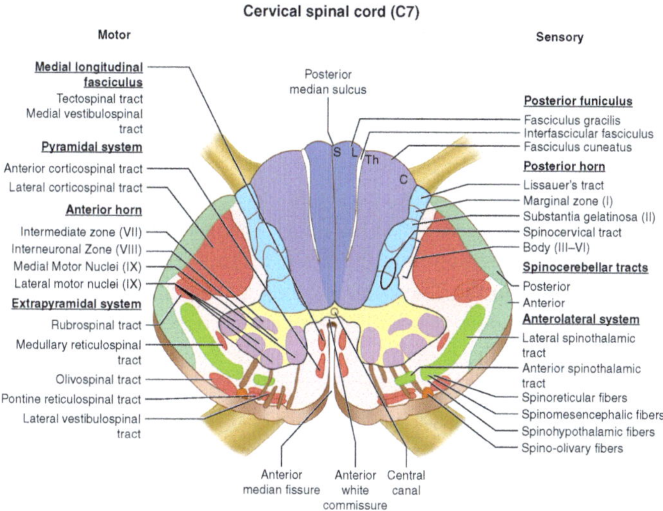

Fig. 1.1 Color-coded transverse section of the cervical spinal cord at C7 illustrating the organization of motor and sensory pathways, laminar zones of the gray matter (Rexed laminae I–IX), anterior horn motor nuclei, posterior funiculus subdivisions (fasciculi gracilis and cuneatus), pyramidal and extrapyramidal descending systems, anterolateral system, spinocerebellar tracts, and the somatotopic arrangement of fibers within the posterior funiculus (sacral, lumbar, thoracic, and cervical from medial to lateral)

distinguished by intermediolateral cell columns housing sympathetic preganglionic neurons.
- *Lumbar region*: Shows decreased white matter but large anterior horn enlargements for motor innervation of the lower limbs; intermediolateral cell columns contain parasympathetic preganglionic neurons; forms the lumbar enlargement.
- *Sacral region*: Exhibits minimal white matter; intermediolateral cell columns persist, containing parasympathetic preganglionic neurons controlling pelvic organs.

External Features

- *Cervical enlargement*: The spinal cord widens at cervical (C5-T1) and lumbar regions to accommodate increased neuronal populations for limb control. The cervical enlargement gives rise to the brachial plexus, which supplies motor and sensory innervation to the upper limbs.
- *Lumbar enlargement*: Corresponds to spinal segments L2-S3 and gives rise to the lumbosacral plexus, which provides comprehensive innervation to the lower limbs.
- *Conus medullaris*: The tapered, conical termination of the spinal cord, located around the L1-L2 vertebral level in adults; injury to this structure produces a distinct clinical syndrome.
- *Cauda equina*: A bundle of spinal nerve roots descending from the conus medullaris, resembling a "horse's tail." These roots extend through the vertebral canal to exit at their appropriate intervertebral foramina; this anatomical arrangement allows for safe lumbar puncture below L2.

Internal Anatomy of the Spinal Cord

Gray Matter Organization

Location and morphology: The gray matter occupies a central position within the spinal cord, appearing in cross section as a butterfly or H-shaped structure. This distinctive configuration consists of two posterior (dorsal) horns, two anterior (ventral) horns, and in thoracic and upper lumbar regions, lateral horns.

Composition: Gray matter comprises neuronal cell bodies, dendrites, synaptic connections, glial cells (astrocytes, oligodendrocytes, microglia), and an extensive capillary network. This region is the primary site of information processing and integration within the spinal cord, including reflex circuits, sensory relay, and motor command execution.

Functional regions:

- *Dorsal (posterior) horns*: Receive sensory (afferent) information from the body via the dorsal roots of spinal nerves. The dorsal horn is organized into distinct laminae (Rexed laminae I–VI), each processing specific sensory modalities including pain, temperature, touch, and proprioception.
- *Ventral (anterior) horns*: Contain the cell bodies of alpha and gamma motor neurons that send efferent signals to skeletal muscles. Alpha motor neurons innervate extrafusal muscle fibers for force generation, while gamma motor neurons control intrafusal muscle spindle sensitivity.
- *Lateral horns*: Present in thoracic (T1-L2) and sacral (S2-S4) regions, these contain autonomic motor neurons. Thoracolumbar lateral horns house sympathetic preganglionic neurons, while sacral lateral horns contain parasympathetic preganglionic neurons.

White Matter Organization

Location and structure: White matter surrounds the central gray matter and consists predominantly of myelinated axons organized into ascending (sensory) and descending (motor) tracts. The myelin sheaths, produced by oligodendrocytes, give this tissue its characteristic white appearance and enable rapid saltatory conduction of action potentials.

Organization into columns: The white matter is divided into three primary columns (funiculi), each containing multiple functionally distinct tracts (fasciculi). Tracts consist of axons with similar origin, destination, and function, forming the anatomical basis for predictable clinical syndromes when damaged.

Major white matter columns:

- *Dorsal (posterior) columns*: Carry ascending sensory information for fine discriminative touch, conscious proprioception, and vibration sense from the body to the brain. Composed of the fasciculus gracilis (lower body) medially and fasciculus cuneatus (upper body) laterally.
- *Lateral columns*: Contain both sensory and motor tracts. The lateral corticospinal tract (pyramidal tract) is particularly prominent, conveying voluntary motor commands from the motor cortex to spinal motor neurons. Also includes the spinocerebellar tracts (unconscious proprioception), spinothalamic tract (pain and temperature), and rubrospinal tract.
- *Ventral (anterior) columns*: Primarily involved in motor control and coordination, including the ventral corticospinal tract, vestibulospinal tract (balance and posture), reticulospinal tract (automatic movement and tone), and tectospinal tract (reflex head movements). Also contains the anterior spinothalamic tract for crude touch and pressure sensation.

Central Canal

Location and structure: The central canal is a cerebrospinal fluid-filled channel running longitudinally through the center of the spinal cord, extending from the fourth ventricle in the brainstem to the conus medullaris. The canal is lined by specialized ependymal cells, which form a barrier between the CSF and neural tissue.

Function: In adults, the central canal is typically small and may become partially or completely obliterated in some regions, though it continues to play a role in CSF circulation and metabolic support of central spinal cord tissue. Pathological expansion of the central canal (hydromyelia) or formation of fluid-filled cavities in the cord parenchyma (syringomyelia) can cause significant neurological deficits.

Spinal Nerves and Root Organization

The spinal cord communicates with the peripheral nervous system through 31 pairs of spinal nerves that exit the vertebral column through the intervertebral foramina. This segmental organization allows precise topographic representation of body regions and forms the anatomical basis for dermatomal and myotomal clinical examination.

Spinal Nerve Composition and Formation

Root components:

- *Dorsal (posterior) root*: Carries sensory (afferent) fibers from the body to the spinal cord. The cell bodies of these pseudounipolar neurons are located in the dorsal root ganglion, positioned just outside the spinal cord within or near the intervertebral foramen.
- *Ventral (anterior) root*: Carries motor (efferent) fibers from the spinal cord to muscles and glands. The cell bodies of these neurons reside in the ventral horn (somatic motor) or lateral horn (autonomic motor) of the spinal cord gray matter.

The dorsal and ventral roots unite to form a mixed spinal nerve containing both sensory and motor fibers. Shortly after formation, each spinal nerve divides into two main branches:

- *Dorsal (posterior) ramus*: Carries sensory and motor fibers to the posterior body wall, including the paraspinal muscles and overlying skin.
- *Ventral (anterior) ramus*: Carries sensory and motor fibers to the anterior and lateral body wall and the limbs; ventral rami form nerve plexuses in cervical, brachial, and lumbosacral regions.

Major Spinal Nerve Plexuses

In cervical, lumbar, and sacral regions, the ventral rami interweave to form nerve plexuses before distributing to peripheral structures. This reorganization allows multiple spinal segments to contribute to individual peripheral nerves, providing functional redundancy and complex innervation patterns.

- *Cervical plexus (C1–C4)*: Provides motor and sensory innervation to the neck and head. Most clinically significant is the phrenic nerve (C3–C5), which innervates the diaphragm; damage above C3 can result in ventilator dependence.
- *Brachial plexus (C5–T1)*: Innervates the upper limb through complex reorganization into trunks, divisions, cords, and branches. Major terminal branches include the musculocutaneous, axillary, radial, median, and ulnar nerves.
- *Lumbar plexus (L1–L4)*: Provides sensory and motor innervation to the anterior and medial thigh, as well as portions of the leg. Major branches include the femoral and obturator nerves.
- *Sacral plexus (L4–S4)*: Supplies the posterior thigh, leg, and foot, as well as pelvic structures. The sciatic nerve, the body's largest nerve, arises from this plexus and divides into the tibial and common fibular nerves.

Functional Organization of the Spinal Cord

The spinal cord serves as both a conduit for information between the brain and body and an independent integrative center. Its functional organization reflects the elegant coordination of sensory input, motor output, reflex circuits, and autonomic control essential for survival and adaptive behavior.

Motor Function

The spinal cord transmits motor commands from the brain to skeletal muscles through descending motor pathways. These pathways are traditionally divided into pyramidal (corticospinal) and extrapyramidal systems, though this distinction is somewhat artificial as these systems extensively interact.

- *Pyramidal tract (corticospinal)*: Originates in the motor cortex and descends through the internal capsule, cerebral peduncles, and medullary pyramids. Approximately 90% of fibers decussate at the pyramids to form the lateral corticospinal tract, controlling fine, voluntary movements of the contralateral limbs.
- *Extrapyramidal tracts*: Include the rubrospinal (limb flexion), vestibulospinal (balance and extensor tone), reticulospinal (automatic movements and muscle tone), and tectospinal (reflex head movements in response to visual stimuli) tracts. These pathways modulate movement, posture, and muscle tone.

Sensory Function

The spinal cord receives diverse sensory information from the body and relays this information to the brain through specialized ascending pathways. Different sensory modalities travel in anatomically distinct tracts, a principle with profound clinical implications.

- *Dorsal column-medial lemniscal pathway*: Conveys fine touch, vibration, conscious proprioception, and two-point discrimination. First-order neurons ascend ipsilaterally in the dorsal columns to the medulla, where they synapse and decussate.
- *Spinothalamic tract (anterolateral system)*: Transmits pain, temperature, and crude touch. First-order neurons synapse in the dorsal horn, and second-order neurons decussate immediately before ascending contralaterally to the thalamus.
- *Spinocerebellar tracts*: Carry unconscious proprioception from muscles, tendons, and joints to the cerebellum for coordination. The dorsal spinocerebellar tract ascends ipsilaterally, while the ventral spinocerebellar tract ascends contralaterally after double-crossing.

Reflex Circuits

The spinal cord executes reflex arcs—automatic, involuntary responses to stimuli that occur without conscious brain involvement. These reflexes serve protective functions and maintain basic motor control. A classic example is the patellar reflex (knee jerk), where stretching the patellar tendon activates muscle spindles in the quadriceps. Sensory neurons convey this information to the spinal cord, which directly activates motor neurons to contract the quadriceps, producing leg extension. Simultaneously, inhibitory interneurons suppress antagonist (hamstring) activity, demonstrating reciprocal innervation.

Autonomic Function

The spinal cord plays a central role in autonomic nervous system function, particularly through the sympathetic and parasympathetic divisions. The thoracolumbar spinal cord (T1–L2) contains sympathetic preganglionic neurons in the intermediolateral cell columns. These neurons regulate heart rate, blood pressure, sweating, gastrointestinal motility, and pupillary dilation. The sacral spinal cord (S2–S4) houses parasympathetic preganglionic neurons controlling bladder, bowel, and sexual function. Spinal cord injury disrupting these autonomic centers can cause profound cardiovascular instability, thermoregulatory dysfunction, and loss of bowel/bladder control.

Essential Anatomical Principles

Bell-Magendie Law

This fundamental principle states that dorsal roots contain primary afferent (sensory) fibers while ventral roots contain primary efferent (motor) fibers. However, exceptions exist: some primary afferent fibers travel in ventral roots, explaining why complete dorsal root sectioning does not eliminate all pain sensation from that segment.

Dorsal Root Ganglia
Located in close proximity to the intervertebral foramina with which they are associated. Compression of a dorsal root ganglion produces characteristic radicular pain in the corresponding dermatome, often described as sharp, shooting, or electric-like and following a predictable anatomical distribution.

Important Functional Nuclei

Specific nuclei within the spinal cord gray matter serve specialized functions and have clinical significance:

- *Phrenic nucleus*: Located in the medial anterior horn from C3 to C5, these motor neurons innervate the diaphragm. Bilateral damage causes respiratory failure; unilateral damage produces hemidiaphragm paralysis.
- *Spinal accessory nucleus*: Located in the lateral posterior portion of the anterior horn (intermediolateral column) extending from the caudal medulla to C5. These neurons contribute to the spinal accessory nerve (CN XI), innervating the trapezius and sternocleidomastoid muscles.
- *Clarke's nucleus (nucleus dorsalis)*: Located medial to the intermediolateral cell column, just anteromedial to the dorsal horn, extending from T1 to L2. This relay nucleus receives proprioceptive information from muscle spindles and Golgi tendon organs and gives rise to the dorsal spinocerebellar tract.
- *Onuf's nucleus*: Located in the ventral horn of the sacral spinal cord (S2-S4), these motor neurons innervate the external urethral and external anal sphincters, providing voluntary control over micturition and defecation.

Major Ascending and Descending Tracts

Understanding the anatomical organization of spinal cord tracts is essential for clinical localization of pathology. Each tract has characteristic location, function, and pattern of decussation (crossing), enabling clinicians to predict specific deficits from focal lesions.

Ascending (Sensory) Tracts

Dorsal Columns (Posterior Columns)

- *Function*: Fine discriminative touch, conscious proprioception, vibration sense.
- *Pathway*: First-order neurons ascend ipsilaterally in fasciculus gracilis (lower body/leg) or fasciculus cuneatus (upper body/arm); synapse in medulla; decussate as internal arcuate fibers; ascend as medial lemniscus.
- *Clinical correlation*: Loss causes ipsilateral loss of vibration and proprioception; positive Romberg sign; sensory ataxia.

Spinothalamic Tract (Anterolateral System)

- *Function*: Pain, temperature, crude touch.
- *Pathway*: First-order neurons synapse in dorsal horn; second-order neurons decussate within one to two segments and ascend contralaterally to the thalamus.
- *Clinical correlation*: Lesion causes contralateral loss of pain and temperature beginning one to two dermatomes below the lesion level.

Spinocerebellar Tracts

- *Function*: Unconscious proprioception for motor coordination.
- *Dorsal spinocerebellar tract*: Ascends ipsilaterally from Clarke's nucleus to inferior cerebellar peduncle; conveys information from lower limb and trunk.
- *Ventral spinocerebellar tract*: Initially crosses, ascends contralaterally, then crosses again in the cerebellum; conveys information from lower limb.
- *Cuneocerebellar tract*: Upper limb equivalent to dorsal spinocerebellar tract; ascends ipsilaterally.

Descending (Motor) Tracts

Lateral Corticospinal Tract

- *Function*: Voluntary movement, particularly fine motor control of extremities.
- *Pathway*: Originates in motor cortex; descends through internal capsule and cerebral peduncles; decussates at medullary pyramids; descends contralaterally.
- *Clinical correlation*: Upper motor neuron lesion causes contralateral weakness, spasticity, hyperreflexia, and Babinski sign.

Anterior Corticospinal Tract

- *Function*: Voluntary movement of axial and proximal limb muscles.
- *Pathway*: Descends ipsilaterally; decussates at spinal segmental level before synapsing.
- *Clinical correlation*: Contributes to bilateral control of trunk musculature.

Extrapyramidal Tracts

- *Rubrospinal tract*: From red nucleus; facilitates flexor muscle tone; crosses in midbrain.
- *Vestibulospinal tracts*: From vestibular nuclei; facilitate extensor muscle tone and balance; mostly ipsilateral.
- *Reticulospinal tracts*: From reticular formation; modulate muscle tone, posture, and locomotion; bilateral.
- *Tectospinal tract*: From superior colliculus; coordinates head and eye movements; crosses in midbrain.

Vascular Supply of the Spinal Cord

The spinal cord receives its blood supply from a complex system of longitudinal and segmental arteries. Understanding this vascular anatomy is crucial for recognizing spinal cord ischemia syndromes and planning surgical interventions.

Arterial Supply

- *Anterior spinal artery*: Formed by branches from both vertebral arteries; descends in the anterior median fissure; supplies the anterior two-thirds of the spinal cord including anterior horns, lateral corticospinal tracts, and spinothalamic tracts. Occlusion produces anterior spinal artery syndrome with motor paralysis and pain/temperature loss, while preserving dorsal column function.
- *Posterior spinal arteries*: Paired arteries arising from vertebral or posterior inferior cerebellar arteries; descend along dorsolateral aspect of spinal cord; supply the posterior one-third including dorsal columns and dorsal horns.
- *Radicular arteries*: Segmental branches from vertebral, cervical, intercostal, lumbar, and sacral arteries that reinforce longitudinal vessels. The artery of Adamkiewicz (great radicular artery) typically arises at T9-L2 and provides crucial blood supply to the lower thoracic and lumbar enlargement.

Venous Drainage

Venous drainage follows a pattern parallel to arterial supply, with anterior and posterior spinal veins draining into radicular veins. These empty into the epidural venous plexus, which communicates with the azygos system and ultimately returns blood to the heart via the superior and inferior vena cavae. This valveless system allows bidirectional flow, creating pathways for metastatic spread from pelvic and thoracic organs.

Vascular Watersheds

The spinal cord contains vulnerable watershed zones between vascular territories, particularly at T1–T4 (where cervical and thoracic blood supply meets) and L1 (where the artery of Adamkiewicz distribution ends). These regions are particularly susceptible to ischemic injury during hypotensive episodes or aortic surgery.

Protective Structures: Meninges and CSF

The spinal cord is protected by three meningeal layers and surrounded by cerebrospinal fluid, providing mechanical cushioning, metabolic support, and immunological surveillance.

Meningeal Layers

- *Dura mater*: The outermost, toughest layer composed of dense collagenous tissue. It forms a tubular sheath extending from the foramen magnum to S2, anchored laterally by denticulate ligaments. The epidural space between dura and vertebral periosteum contains fat, connective tissue, and the internal vertebral venous plexus.
- *Arachnoid mater*: A delicate, avascular membrane closely applied to the inner surface of the dura. The subarachnoid space beneath it contains CSF and the major blood vessels supplying the spinal cord.
- *Pia mater*: The innermost layer intimately adhering to the spinal cord surface, following all contours including the anterior median fissure and posterolateral sulci. Lateral extensions form the denticulate ligaments that anchor the cord.

Cerebrospinal Fluid

CSF is produced primarily by the choroid plexus in the brain ventricles and circulates through the ventricular system before entering the subarachnoid space. The spinal subarachnoid space communicates freely with the cranial subarachnoid space, allowing CSF sampling via lumbar puncture below the conus medullaris (usually L3–L4 or L4–L5). Normal CSF contains few cells, minimal protein, and approximately two-thirds the glucose concentration of blood.

Embryological Development

Understanding spinal cord development illuminates both normal anatomy and congenital malformations. The spinal cord develops from the neural tube, which forms during the third week of embryonic development through neurulation.

Neurulation and Neural Tube Formation

The neural plate, derived from ectoderm, folds to form the neural groove, which then closes to create the neural tube. Closure begins in the cervical region and proceeds both cranially and caudally. Failure of neural tube closure results in neural tube defects such as spina bifida (incomplete posterior closure) or anencephaly (incomplete anterior closure). Folic acid supplementation during pregnancy significantly reduces neural tube defect risk.

Differential Growth and Ascent

During fetal development, the vertebral column grows faster than the spinal cord, causing the apparent "ascent" of the cord relative to the vertebrae. At birth, the spinal cord typically ends at L3; by adulthood, it ends at L1–L2. This differential growth explains why spinal nerve roots must travel increasingly oblique courses to reach their corresponding intervertebral foramina, forming the cauda equina below the conus medullaris.

Gray and White Matter Differentiation

Within the developing neural tube, cells in the ventricular zone proliferate and migrate to form distinct regions. The alar plate (dorsal) gives rise to sensory structures (dorsal horns), while the basal plate (ventral) forms motor structures (ventral horns). The white matter develops later as axons grow along established pathways, with myelination continuing into early childhood.

Clinical Correlations and Spinal Cord Syndromes

Knowledge of spinal cord anatomy enables precise localization of pathology and prediction of clinical manifestations. Understanding these correlations is essential for neurological diagnosis and management.

Traumatic Spinal Cord Injury

Complete Transection

- *Mechanism*: Usually results from severe trauma such as motor vehicle accidents, falls, or penetrating injuries.
- *Clinical features*: Complete loss of motor function, sensation, and reflexes below the injury level. Initial spinal shock with flaccid paralysis and areflexia transitions to spastic paralysis with hyperreflexia over weeks to months.
- *Associated dysfunction*: Bowel and bladder incontinence, sexual dysfunction, loss of temperature regulation, orthostatic hypotension (particularly with cervical and high thoracic injuries affecting sympathetic outflow).

Brown-Séquard Syndrome (Hemisection)

- *Mechanism*: Lateral hemisection of the spinal cord, most commonly from penetrating trauma or tumor.
- *Ipsilateral findings*: Motor paralysis (lateral corticospinal tract), loss of vibration and proprioception (dorsal columns), hyperreflexia and Babinski sign below lesion.
- *Contralateral findings*: Loss of pain and temperature sensation beginning one to two segments below the lesion (spinothalamic tract).

Central Cord Syndrome

- *Mechanism*: Hyperextension injury in patients with pre-existing cervical stenosis; disproportionate damage to central gray matter and medial white matter.

- *Clinical features*: Greater motor impairment in upper extremities than lower extremities (reflecting somatotopic organization of lateral corticospinal tract); variable sensory loss; often spares sacral sensation due to peripheral location of sacral tracts.
- *Prognosis*: Best prognosis among incomplete spinal cord injury syndromes; significant recovery possible with appropriate rehabilitation.

Anterior Cord Syndrome

- *Mechanism*: Damage to anterior two-thirds of spinal cord, typically from anterior spinal artery occlusion.
- *Clinical features*: Motor paralysis (corticospinal tracts), loss of pain and temperature sensation (spinothalamic tracts); preservation of proprioception and vibration (dorsal columns spared).
- *Prognosis*: Generally poor for motor recovery.

Posterior Cord Syndrome

- *Mechanism*: Rare; selective damage to dorsal columns from posterior spinal artery occlusion, demyelination, or dorsal column degeneration.
- *Clinical features*: Loss of proprioception and vibration sense; preserved motor function and pain/temperature sensation; severe sensory ataxia and positive Romberg sign.

Conus Medullaris vs. Cauda Equina Syndrome

Conus medullaris syndrome: Injury to the terminal spinal cord at L1–L2; presents with bilateral symmetric lower extremity weakness, early bowel/bladder dysfunction (areflexic), saddle anesthesia, and mixed upper and lower motor neuron signs.

Cauda equina syndrome: Compression of lumbosacral nerve roots below the conus; presents with asymmetric lower extremity weakness, late bowel/bladder dysfunction, radicular pain, and pure lower motor neuron signs (flaccid paralysis, areflexia). Typically requires urgent surgical decompression.

Degenerative and Demyelinating Disorders

Amyotrophic Lateral Sclerosis (ALS)

- *Pathophysiology*: Progressive neurodegenerative disease affecting both upper motor neurons (brain) and lower motor neurons (spinal cord anterior horns), with characteristic sparing of extraocular muscles and sensory systems.
- *Clinical features*: Muscle weakness and atrophy beginning focally, usually in limbs, with eventual spread to bulbar and respiratory muscles. Combination of upper motor neuron signs (spasticity, hyperreflexia) and lower motor neuron signs (atrophy, fasciculations).
- *Prognosis*: Progressive disease with median survival of 3–5 years from symptom onset; respiratory failure is typical cause of death.

Multiple Sclerosis (MS)

- *Pathophysiology*: Autoimmune demyelinating disease targeting myelin sheaths in the CNS; characterized by inflammatory plaques (demyelinated areas) disseminated in space and time.
- *Spinal cord involvement*: Common site of MS plaques; can affect any spinal tract, producing diverse symptoms including spasticity, weakness, sensory disturbances (particularly posterior column dysfunction), bladder/bowel dysfunction, and Lhermitte's sign (electric shock sensation with neck flexion).
- *Clinical course*: Most commonly relapsing-remitting pattern with acute exacerbations followed by partial or complete recovery; may progress to secondary progressive disease.

Spinal Muscular Atrophy (SMA)

- *Pathophysiology*: Genetic disorder caused by SMN1 gene mutations leading to degeneration of lower motor neurons in spinal cord anterior horns; classified into Types 1–4 based on age of onset and severity.
- *Clinical features*: Progressive symmetric muscle weakness and atrophy; Type 1 (Werdnig-Hoffmann disease) presents in infancy with severe weakness, hypotonia, and respiratory compromise; later-onset types show milder, slower progression.

- *Treatment advances*: Gene therapy and SMN2-targeted therapies have dramatically improved outcomes, particularly when initiated early.

Inflammatory Disorders

Transverse Myelitis

- *Pathophysiology*: Acute inflammatory disorder affecting a focal segment of spinal cord, causing demyelination and axonal damage across one or more spinal levels.
- *Etiology*: Idiopathic in many cases; may be associated with viral infections, vaccination, MS, neuromyelitis optica, or systemic autoimmune diseases.
- *Clinical presentation*: Rapid onset (hours to days) of bilateral motor weakness, sensory loss at a defined level, pain, bladder/bowel dysfunction, and muscle spasms.
- *Treatment*: High-dose corticosteroids, plasma exchange for refractory cases; outcomes variable ranging from complete recovery to permanent disability.

Neuromyelitis Optica Spectrum Disorder (NMOSD)

- *Pathophysiology*: Autoimmune disorder characterized by antibodies against aquaporin-4 water channels, predominantly affecting optic nerves and spinal cord.
- *Clinical features*: Severe optic neuritis (often bilateral) with significant vision loss, longitudinally extensive transverse myelitis ($\geq$3 vertebral segments), intractable nausea/hiccups from area postrema involvement.
- *Distinction from MS*: Spinal cord lesions longer and more severe than typical MS; positive anti-aquaporin-4 antibodies; different treatment approach requiring immunosuppression rather than MS disease-modifying therapies.

Vascular Disorders

Spinal Cord Ischemia and Infarction

- *Etiology*: Arterial occlusion (thrombosis, embolism), hypoperfusion, aortic dissection or surgery, vasculitis, or compression of radicular arteries.
- *Anterior spinal artery syndrome*: Most common pattern; sudden onset of flaccid paralysis progressing to spastic paralysis, loss of pain and temperature sensation bilaterally, with preserved proprioception and vibration (dorsal columns spared).
- *Clinical presentation*: Acute onset of bilateral weakness and sensory loss, often with pain at the level of ischemia. In severe cases, autonomic dysfunction including hypotension and bladder/bowel incontinence.
- *High-risk scenarios*: Thoracoabdominal aortic surgery, prolonged hypotension, aortic dissection, atherosclerotic disease of radicular arteries.

Spinal Hemorrhage

- *Types*: Epidural hematoma (between dura and vertebrae), subdural hematoma (between dura and arachnoid), subarachnoid hemorrhage, or intramedullary (within cord parenchyma).
- *Causes*: Arteriovenous malformations, anticoagulation, trauma, bleeding disorders, or spontaneous.
- *Clinical presentation*: Sudden severe back or neck pain, rapid progression of neurological deficits including weakness, sensory loss, and bowel/bladder dysfunction.
- *Treatment*: Often requires urgent surgical decompression for epidural or subdural hematomas.

Infectious Disorders

Spinal Epidural Abscess

- *Pathophysiology*: Bacterial infection (most commonly *Staphylococcus aureus*) in the epidural space causing spinal cord compression through direct pressure and vascular compromise.

- *Risk factors*: Diabetes, immunosuppression, IV drug use, spinal procedures or surgery, bacteremia from distant infection.
- *Clinical presentation*: Classic triad of fever, back pain, and neurological deficits, though complete triad present in minority. Progressive symptoms through stages: back pain → radicular pain → weakness → paralysis.
- *Treatment*: Medical emergency requiring prompt IV antibiotics and often urgent surgical drainage; prognosis depends heavily on timing of intervention.

Tuberculosis of the Spine (Pott's Disease)

- *Pathophysiology*: Mycobacterium tuberculosis infection spreading hematogenously to vertebral bodies, causing destruction, collapse, and potential spinal cord compromise.
- *Clinical features*: Insidious onset of back pain, spinal deformity (gibbus deformity—sharp angulation from vertebral collapse), constitutional symptoms (fever, night sweats, weight loss), and variable neurological deficits.
- *Diagnosis*: MRI shows vertebral destruction with paravertebral soft tissue masses; tissue biopsy for culture and histology essential for confirmation.
- *Treatment*: Prolonged anti-tuberculosis therapy (6–12 months); surgery for significant deformity or neurological compromise.

Structural and Compressive Disorders

Spinal Stenosis

- *Pathophysiology*: Narrowing of the spinal canal, lateral recesses, or neural foramina causing compression of spinal cord or nerve roots.
- *Causes*: Degenerative changes (most common)—facet joint hypertrophy, ligamentum flavum thickening, disc bulging, osteophyte formation. Less commonly: congenital, spondylolisthesis, trauma.

- *Clinical features*: Neurogenic claudication (leg pain, weakness, numbness with walking, relieved by rest and flexion), back pain, radicular symptoms. Cervical stenosis may cause myelopathy with gait dysfunction and upper extremity weakness.
- *Treatment*: Conservative management initially; surgical decompression for progressive myelopathy or refractory symptoms.

Herniated Intervertebral Disc

- *Pathophysiology*: Displacement of nucleus pulposus through tears in the annulus fibrosus, causing compression of adjacent nerve roots or, less commonly, the spinal cord.
- *Common levels*: L4–L5 and L5–S1 most frequent in lumbar spine; C5–C6 and C6–C7 in cervical spine.
- *Clinical presentation*: Radicular pain (sciatica in lumbar disc herniation), dermatomal sensory loss, myotomal weakness, reduced reflexes. Central disc herniation may cause cauda equina syndrome (surgical emergency).
- *Treatment*: Most cases resolve with conservative management; surgery reserved for cauda equina syndrome, progressive weakness, or refractory pain.

Syringomyelia

- *Pathophysiology*: Formation of a fluid-filled cavity (syrinx) within the spinal cord parenchyma, most commonly in the cervical region.
- *Causes*: Chiari malformation (most common), trauma, tumors, arachnoiditis, or idiopathic.
- *Clinical features*: Classic "cape-like" distribution of pain and temperature loss over shoulders and upper back (spinothalamic tract damage at syrinx level), with preserved light touch (dorsal columns intact). Progressive weakness and atrophy of hands, scoliosis.
- *Treatment*: Surgical decompression and syrinx drainage; treatment of underlying cause when identified.

Neoplastic Disorders

Classification of Spinal Tumors

Spinal tumors are classified by location relative to the dura and spinal cord:

- *Extradural (55%)*: Outside the dura; most commonly metastases from breast, lung, prostate, kidney, or thyroid cancer. Also includes vertebral body tumors.
- *Intradural-extramedullary (40%)*: Within the dura but outside the cord; most commonly meningiomas and nerve sheath tumors (schwannomas, neurofibromas).
- *Intramedullary (5%)*: Within the spinal cord parenchyma; most commonly ependymomas and astrocytomas.

Primary Intramedullary Tumors

- *Ependymomas*: Most common primary intramedullary tumor in adults; arise from ependymal cells lining central canal; typically well-circumscribed; often in cervical or thoracic regions; may be amenable to complete surgical resection.
- *Astrocytomas*: Second most common; more infiltrative than ependymomas making complete resection challenging; more common in children; variable grade and prognosis.
- *Clinical presentation*: Insidious onset of pain (often at night), progressive weakness, sensory disturbances, and bowel/bladder dysfunction. Central cord syndrome pattern may develop.

Metastatic Spinal Tumors

- *Epidemiology*: Most common malignant spinal tumors; present in up to 70% of cancer patients at autopsy; often first manifestation of occult malignancy.
- *Clinical features*: Severe, progressive back pain (worse at night and with recumbency), rapid neurological deterioration possible. Pathological fracture may cause acute spinal cord compression.
- *Treatment*: Depends on tumor type, extent, patient prognosis, and neurological status. Options include radiation therapy, sur-

gery, chemotherapy, or combination approaches. Spinal cord compression is an oncological emergency requiring urgent treatment.

Conclusion

The spinal cord represents a remarkably organized structure whose anatomy directly reflects its diverse functions in motor control, sensory processing, autonomic regulation, and reflex coordination. Mastery of spinal cord neuroanatomy provides the foundation for clinical reasoning in neurology and neurosurgery, enabling precise localization of pathology and prediction of clinical deficits. The integration of gross anatomy, microscopic organization, tract anatomy, vascular supply, and embryological development creates a comprehensive framework for understanding both normal neurological function and the pathophysiology of spinal cord disorders. This knowledge translates directly to clinical practice, informing diagnostic approaches, surgical planning, and therapeutic strategies while emphasizing the critical importance of early recognition and treatment of spinal cord pathology to optimize neurological outcomes.

The Brainstem

2

Introduction

The brainstem is an evolutionarily ancient and structurally complex region of the central nervous system (CNS) that functions as the critical interface between higher brain centers and the spinal cord. This relatively small but extraordinarily important structure controls many vital autonomic functions essential for survival, including respiration, cardiovascular regulation, blood pressure maintenance, and consciousness. Additionally, the brainstem serves as the origin site for ten of the twelve cranial nerves (CN III through XII) and contains the major ascending sensory and descending motor pathways that connect the brain with the rest of the body (Fig. 2.1).

The brainstem can be anatomically divided into three main regions, arranged rostrocaudally (from top to bottom): the midbrain (mesencephalon), the pons (metencephalon), and the

V. Yanamadala, *Essential Neuroanatomy*,
https://doi.org/10.1007/978-3-032-26877-8_2

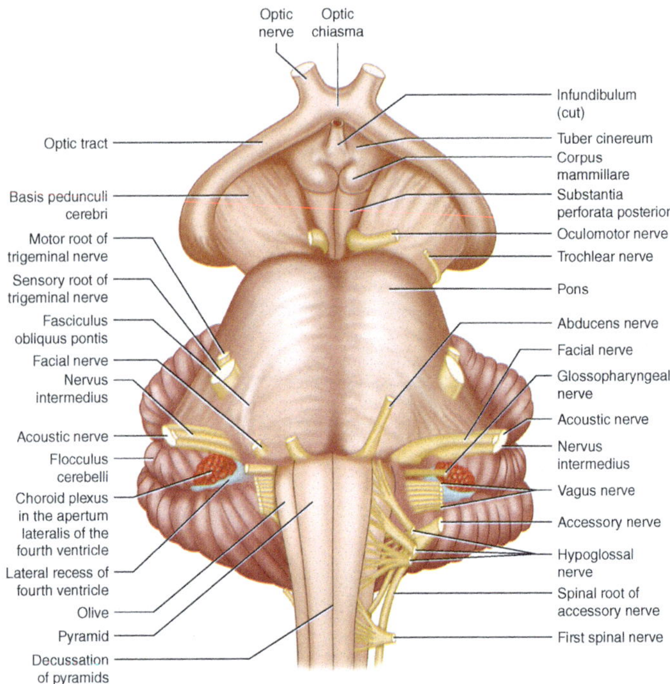

Fig. 2.1 Ventral (inferior) surface of the brainstem and diencephalon showing the origins of cranial nerves II through XII, the optic chiasma, optic tract, infundibulum, tuber cinereum, corpus mamillare (mammillary body), substantia perforata posterior, and major surface landmarks of the pons and medulla oblongata

medulla oblongata (myelencephalon). Each region has distinct structural features, contains specific cranial nerve nuclei, and serves unique physiological functions while maintaining integrated communication between all levels of the nervous system. Understanding the three-dimensional organization and functional

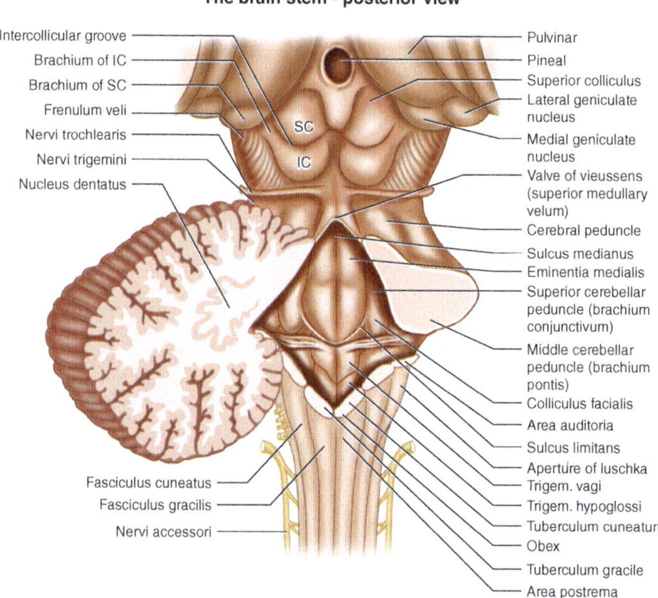

Fig. 2.2 Posterior view of the brainstem with the cerebellum partially retracted, showing the dorsal surface structures of the midbrain, pons, and medulla, including the colliculi, cerebellar peduncles, rhomboid fossa landmarks, and posterior column nuclei and fasciculi

anatomy of the brainstem is essential for clinical neuroscience, as even small lesions in this region can produce profound and life-threatening neurological deficits. Figure 2.2 shows a posterior view of the brain stem, while Fig. 2.3 shows an anteroinferior view of the brainstem and Fig. 2.4 shows a posterolateral view of the brainstem.

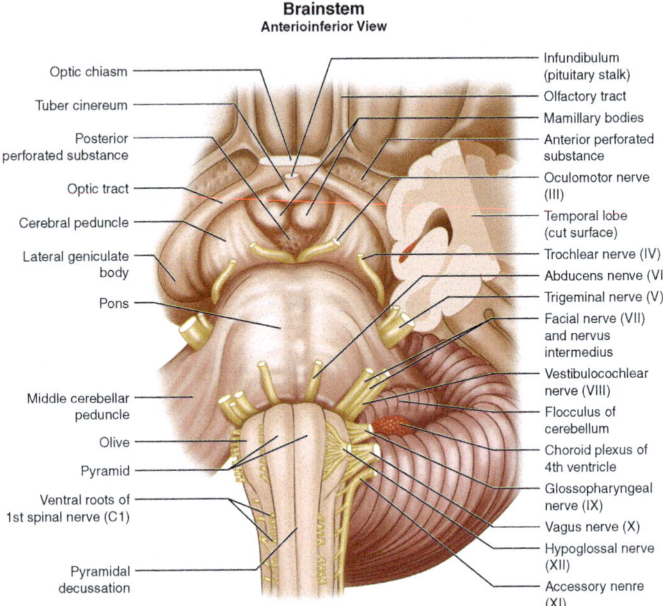

Fig. 2.3 Anteroinferior view of the brainstem illustrating the cranial nerve roots (CN I–XII), brainstem surface anatomy including the cerebral peduncles, pons, olive, pyramid, and associated structures such as the flocculus and choroid plexus of the fourth ventricle

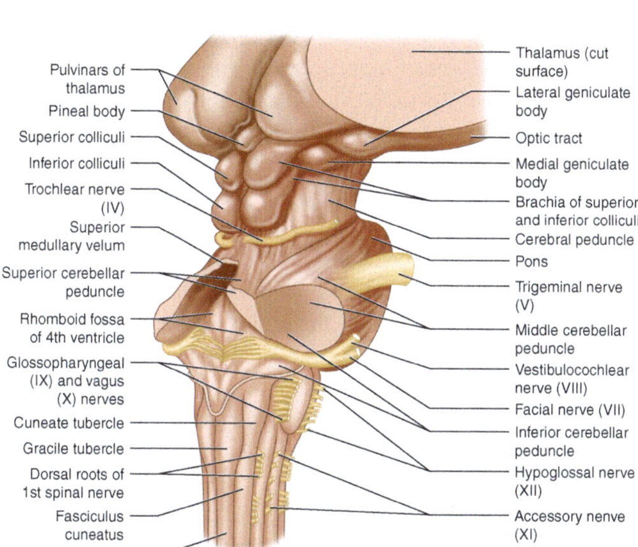

Fig. 2.4 Posterolateral view of the brainstem showing the dorsal and lateral surfaces of the midbrain, pons, and medulla, with identification of the cranial nerve roots, cerebellar peduncles, geniculate bodies, colliculi and their brachia, and posterior column fasciculi

The Midbrain (Mesencephalon)

The midbrain, or mesencephalon, represents the most rostral (uppermost) component of the brainstem. Located immediately caudal to the diencephalon (specifically beneath the thalamus and hypothalamus) and rostral to the pons, the midbrain plays crucial roles in motor movement coordination, visual and auditory processing, arousal, and alertness. The midbrain extends approximately 1.5–2.0 cm in length and surrounds the cerebral aqueduct (aqueduct of Sylvius), a narrow channel that connects the third ventricle with the fourth ventricle, allowing cerebrospinal fluid circulation.

Anatomical Organization of the Midbrain

The midbrain is traditionally divided into three main regions: the tectum (roof), the tegmentum (floor), and the cerebral peduncles (basis pedunculi). This tripartite organization reflects both developmental origins and functional specialization, with each region containing distinct nuclear groups and fiber pathways.

The Tectum

The tectum (Latin for "roof") constitutes the dorsal portion of the midbrain, located posterior to the cerebral aqueduct. The tectum contains four prominent rounded elevations collectively known as the corpora quadrigemina ("quadrigeminal bodies"), which include the paired superior colliculi rostrally and the paired inferior colliculi caudally. These structures are phylogenetically ancient and serve as important sensory processing and reflex centers.

Superior Colliculi

The superior colliculi are multilayered structures that serve as primary centers for visual reflex coordination and visuomotor integration. These nuclei receive direct retinal input via retinotectal fibers from the optic tracts, which travel through the superior brachium. The superior colliculi are particularly important for detecting the direction and velocity of moving objects in the visual field and generating appropriate saccadic eye movements (rapid eye movements) to track these objects. Corticotectal fibers from the frontal eye fields (Brodmann area 8) project to the superior colliculi and vertical gaze centers through the superior brachium, enabling voluntary control of saccades and vertical gaze movements. The superior colliculi also project to the ipsilateral pulvinar and lateral geniculate nucleus of the thalamus via tectothalamic fibers, contributing to visual attention and awareness.

Inferior Colliculi

The inferior colliculi represent the major brainstem auditory relay nuclei and are essential components of the ascending auditory pathway. These structures receive tonotopically organized input from the cochlear nuclei (both dorsal and ventral divisions) and the superior olivary nucleus via the lateral lemniscus. The inferior colliculi contain both spatial maps for sound localization and tonotopic maps that preserve frequency organization from the cochlea. Each inferior colliculus can be subdivided into a central nucleus and a pericentral nucleus, each serving distinct auditory processing functions. Output from the inferior colliculi projects via the inferior brachium to the medial geniculate nucleus (MGN) of the thalamus, which then relays auditory information to the primary auditory cortex. The inferior colliculi also send projections to the superior colliculi to coordinate audiovisual spatial maps and project back to the superior olivary complex to modulate early auditory processing.

The Tegmentum

The tegmentum comprises the ventral region of the midbrain, located anterior to the cerebral aqueduct and posterior to the cerebral peduncles. This region contains numerous functionally diverse nuclei and fiber tracts that are critical for motor control, pain modulation, and arousal.

Red Nucleus

The red nucleus (nucleus ruber) is a prominent iron-rich structure in the midbrain tegmentum that derives its name from its reddish appearance in fresh tissue, attributed to its high iron content and rich vascularization. This nucleus can be divided into two functionally distinct components. The magnocellular (large-celled) part, which is relatively smaller in humans compared to other mammals, gives rise to the rubrospinal tract. This tract receives input from the cerebellar interposed nuclei and plays a role in motor coordination, particularly influencing flexor muscle tone of the upper and lower limbs. The parvocellular (small-celled) part, which is proportionally larger in humans, receives input from the cerebellar dentate nucleus and gives rise to rubroolivary fibers that project to the inferior olivary nuclear complex. These connections are important for motor learning and fine motor control.

Substantia Nigra

The substantia nigra ("black substance") is a large, darkly pigmented nucleus located in the ventral midbrain tegmentum. Its dark appearance results from neuromelanin, a polymer formed during dopamine synthesis in its neurons. The substantia nigra is subdivided into two functionally and neurochemically distinct zones. The pars compacta (compact part) contains densely packed dopaminergic neurons that project throughout the striatum (caudate nucleus and putamen), forming the nigrostriatal pathway. These dopaminergic projections modulate striatal activity and are essential for the initiation and smooth execution of voluntary movements. Degeneration of the pars compacta dopaminergic neurons is the primary pathological hallmark of Parkinson's disease, resulting in the characteristic motor symptoms of tremor, rigidity, bradykinesia, and postural instability. The pars reticulata (reticular part) contains GABAergic neurons and essentially represents a continuation of the internal segment of the globus pallidus. These neurons serve as a major output nucleus of the basal ganglia, projecting to the thalamus and superior colliculus to influence motor control and eye movements.

Periaqueductal Gray

The periaqueductal gray (PAG), also called the central gray, surrounds the cerebral aqueduct throughout the midbrain. This region plays crucial roles in pain modulation, vocalization, reproductive behavior, and defensive behaviors including aggression. The PAG is a key component of the endogenous pain control system, receiving nociceptive information from the spinothalamic tract and modulating pain transmission through descending projections to the rostral ventromedial medulla, which in turn projects to the spinal cord dorsal horn. The PAG also coordinates autonomic and somatic responses to stress and threat, making it essential for survival behaviors.

The Cerebral Peduncles

The cerebral peduncles (crura cerebri) are two large cylindrical bundles of descending nerve fibers located on the anterior (ventral) surface of the midbrain. Each cerebral peduncle contains approximately 21 million fibers, representing one of the largest fiber bundles in the human nervous system. These fibers originate from the cerebral cortex and descend through the internal capsule before entering the cerebral peduncles.

The cerebral peduncles are organized in a characteristic medial-to-lateral arrangement:

- Medial region: Frontopontine fibers originating from the frontal cortex.
- Medial-intermediate region: Corticobulbar fibers destined for cranial nerve nuclei.
- Central region: Corticospinal tract fibers (approximately one million per side) that will form the pyramidal tract and eventually cross at the pyramidal decussation.
- Lateral region: Occipitopontine, parietopontine, and temporopontine fibers from the posterior cortical areas.

The vast majority of cerebral peduncle fibers (approximately 12 million per side) terminate in the ipsilateral pontine nuclei in the basis pontis. Several million additional fibers project to the reticular formation or cranial nerve nuclei. Only about one million fibers per side continue into the ipsilateral pyramid to eventually form the corticospinal tract that controls voluntary movement.

Additional Midbrain Nuclei

Beyond the major structures described above, the midbrain contains several smaller but functionally important nuclei:

Interstitial Nucleus of Cajal (INC)

This nucleus is involved in vertical gaze modulation and works in conjunction with the rostral interstitial nucleus of the medial longitudinal fasciculus (riMLF). The INC also contributes to smooth pursuit eye movements and receives input from the vestibular nuclei via the medial longitudinal fasciculus.

Interpeduncular Nucleus
Located in the interpeduncular fossa between the cerebral peduncles, this nucleus receives major cholinergic input from the habenula (predominantly the medial habenular nucleus) via the fasciculus retroflexus, also known as the habenulointerpeduncular tract. This pathway is important in visceral functions, emotional responses, and behavioral regulation. The interpeduncular nucleus sends output to the hypothalamus via the medial forebrain bundle.

Pedunculopontine Nucleus (PPN)
The pedunculopontine nucleus is a cholinergic nucleus located at the junction of the midbrain and pons. It sends cholinergic fibers to the cerebellum and plays multifaceted roles in motor control, arousal, attention, and cognition. The PPN is an important component of the ascending reticular activating system (ARAS), which maintains consciousness and arousal. It also contributes to the reticulospinal tract and serves as an important relay center for basal ganglia output. The PPN has been implicated in the pathophysiology of Parkinson's disease, particularly regarding gait disturbances and postural instability. The closely associated peripeduncular nucleus shares similar functions and connections.

Parabigeminal Nucleus
This small cholinergic nucleus is located between the two inferior colliculi. It receives input from and projects to the superior colliculi bilaterally, playing a role in visual processing and attention to visual stimuli.

Nucleus of Darkschewitsch
This nucleus projects to nuclei of the posterior commissure and participates in vertical gaze control mechanisms.

Cranial Nerves Originating from the Midbrain

The midbrain gives rise to two cranial nerves that are critical for eye movements:

Oculomotor Nerve (Cranial Nerve III)

The oculomotor nerve nucleus is located in the midbrain tegmentum at the level of the superior colliculus, ventral to the periaqueductal gray. This nerve innervates most of the extraocular muscles, including the superior rectus, inferior rectus, medial rectus, and inferior oblique muscles. The oculomotor nerve also carries parasympathetic fibers from the Edinger-Westphal nucleus, which control pupillary constriction and accommodation for near vision. Damage to CN III results in ptosis (drooping eyelid), dilated pupil, and inability to move the eye upward, downward, or medially.

Trochlear Nerve (Cranial Nerve IV)

The trochlear nerve nucleus is located in the midbrain tegmentum at the level of the inferior colliculus. CN IV is unique among cranial nerves in that it exits from the dorsal surface of the brainstem and is the only cranial nerve that completely decussates. It innervates the superior oblique muscle, which depresses and intorts the eye. Lesions of CN IV cause difficulty looking downward and inward, particularly noticeable when descending stairs or reading.

The Pons

The pons (Latin for "bridge") is the middle segment of the brainstem, situated between the midbrain rostrally and the medulla oblongata caudally. As its name suggests, the pons serves as a crucial bridge connecting the cerebral cortex with the cerebellum and spinal cord. The pons measures approximately 2.5 cm in length and can be divided into two main regions: the ventral basis pontis (basal pons) and the dorsal pontine tegmentum. The pons plays essential roles in respiratory control, sleep-wake cycle regulation, motor coordination, and sensory relay. The upper pons is displayed in Fig. 2.5, while the mid-pons is displayed in Fig. 2.6 and the caudal pons in Fig. 2.7.

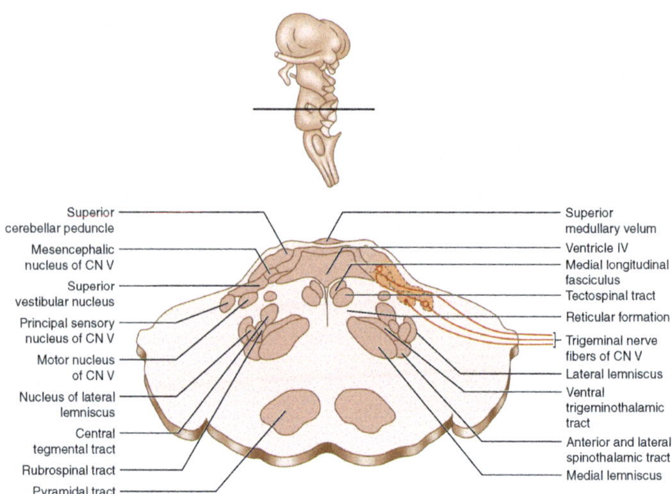

Fig. 2.5 Transverse section through the rostral pons at the level of the trigeminal nerve entry (indicated by a locator diagram), showing the principal sensory and motor nuclei of CN V, the mesencephalic nucleus of CN V, superior vestibular nucleus, nucleus of the lateral lemniscus, superior cerebellar peduncle, superior medullary velum, and major ascending and descending tracts including the medial lemniscus, lateral lemniscus, central tegmental tract, and pyramidal tract

Anatomical Features of the Pons

Pontine Nuclei and Cerebellar Connections

The basis pontis contains the pontine nuclei, which are large collections of neurons (approximately 12 million neurons on each side) that receive massive input from the cerebral cortex via corticopontine fibers. These nuclei process cortical information and relay it to the cerebellum via the middle cerebellar peduncles

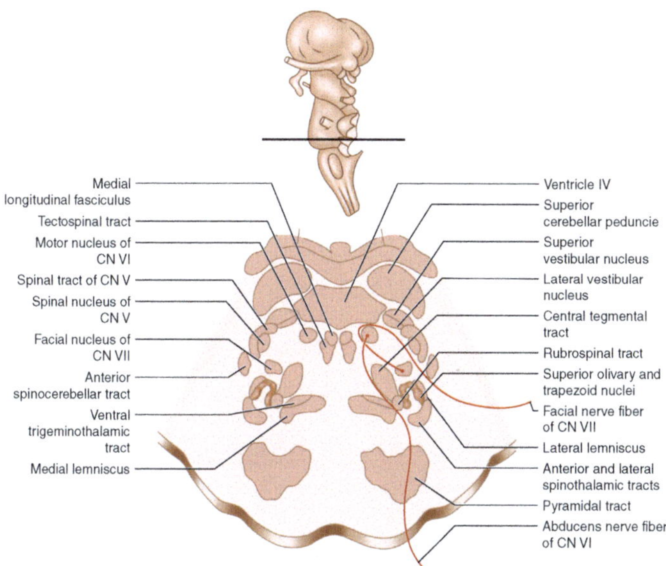

Fig. 2.6 Transverse section through the mid-pons at the level of the facial nucleus and motor nucleus of CN VI (indicated by a locator diagram), showing the superior cerebellar peduncle, vestibular nuclei, lateral lemniscus, superior olivary and trapezoid nuclei, facial nucleus, abducens nerve fibers, central tegmental tract, and major ascending and descending tracts

(brachia pontis), which are the largest of the three cerebellar peduncle pairs. This corticopontocerebellar pathway is crucial for motor planning, coordination, and motor learning. Each middle cerebellar peduncle contains approximately 20 million fibers that cross the midline to enter the contralateral cerebellar hemisphere.

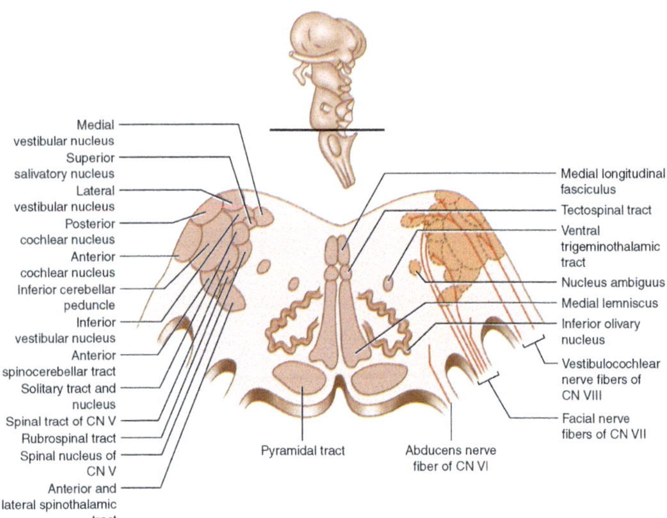

Fig. 2.7 Transverse section through the caudal pons at the level of the facial colliculus (indicated by a locator diagram), showing the abducens and facial nerve nuclei and fibers, cochlear and vestibular nuclei, inferior cerebellar peduncle, and major tracts including the medial lemniscus, pyramidal tract, and spinothalamic tracts

Pontine Respiratory Centers

The pontine tegmentum contains important respiratory control centers, including the pneumotaxic center (also known as the pontine respiratory group) located in the upper pons near the parabrachial nucleus, and the apneustic center in the lower pons. The pneumotaxic center modulates the respiratory rhythm generated by the medullary respiratory centers, particularly by limiting inspiration duration and increasing respiratory rate. The apneustic center promotes inspiration and appears to be involved in gasping respirations. These centers work in coordination with the medullary respiratory centers to maintain appropriate breathing patterns under various physiological conditions.

Locus Coeruleus

The locus coeruleus (LC), also designated as the A6 cell group, is a small but functionally significant nucleus located in the dorsal pontine tegmentum near the floor of the fourth ventricle. The LC is the brain's primary source of norepinephrine (noradrenaline) and contains approximately 15,000–50,000 neurons (with considerable individual variation). Despite its small size, the LC projects extensively throughout the entire central nervous system, including all regions of the cerebral cortex, cerebellum, thalamus, and brainstem. These widespread projections are unique in that they reach the cerebral cortex directly without synapsing in the thalamus, unlike most ascending systems. The LC plays crucial roles in maintaining attention, vigilance, arousal, and the stress response. Its activity increases in response to novel, unexpected, or potentially threatening stimuli, and it receives input from pain pathways. Notably, the LC does not project to the striatum. The surrounding pontine reticular formation also contains additional noradrenergic neurons that project to the spinal cord and modulate motor and autonomic functions.

Cranial Nerves Originating from the Pons

Four cranial nerves emerge from the pons, providing motor, sensory, and autonomic innervation to structures of the head and neck:

Trigeminal Nerve (Cranial Nerve V)

CN V is the largest cranial nerve and provides sensory innervation to the face, oral cavity, nasal cavity, and dura mater, as well as motor innervation to the muscles of mastication. The trigeminal nerve has three major divisions: ophthalmic (V1), maxillary (V2), and mandibular (V3). The trigeminal nuclear complex extends throughout the brainstem from the midbrain to the upper cervical spinal cord and includes the mesencephalic nucleus (proprioception), the main sensory nucleus (discriminative touch), the spinal nucleus (pain and temperature), and the motor nucleus (muscles of mastication).

Abducens Nerve (Cranial Nerve VI)
The abducens nucleus is located in the dorsal pons beneath the facial colliculus in the floor of the fourth ventricle. CN VI innervates the lateral rectus muscle, which abducts the eye (moves it laterally away from the midline). The abducens nucleus contains not only motor neurons that innervate the lateral rectus muscle but also interneurons whose axons decussate and ascend in the contralateral medial longitudinal fasciculus (MLF) to reach the medial rectus subnucleus of the oculomotor nucleus. This connection coordinates conjugate horizontal gaze movements.

Facial Nerve (Cranial Nerve VII)
The facial nerve provides motor innervation to the muscles of facial expression, carries taste sensation from the anterior two-thirds of the tongue, and provides parasympathetic innervation to the lacrimal, submandibular, and sublingual glands. The facial motor nucleus is located in the ventrolateral pontine tegmentum. The facial nerve fibers loop around the abducens nucleus, creating the internal genu before emerging from the brainstem at the pontomedullary junction.

Vestibulocochlear Nerve (Cranial Nerve VIII)
CN VIII has two functional components: the cochlear division for hearing and the vestibular division for balance and spatial orientation. The cochlear nuclei (dorsal and ventral) are located at the pontomedullary junction and receive input from the spiral ganglion of the cochlea. The vestibular nuclear complex, consisting of four main nuclei (superior, medial, lateral, and inferior), extends from the pons into the rostral medulla and receives input from the vestibular apparatus of the inner ear.

The Medulla Oblongata

The medulla oblongata, commonly called simply the medulla, is the most caudal segment of the brainstem. It extends from the pons superiorly to the spinal cord inferiorly, with the transition typically occurring at the level of the foramen magnum or the first cervical vertebra. The medulla measures approximately 3 cm in length and can be divided into a rostral (open) portion where the fourth ventricle is visible dorsally, and a caudal (closed) portion where the central canal is surrounded by neural tissue. The medulla contains numerous vital centers for autonomic regulation and serves as the conduit for major ascending and descending pathways. The mid-medulla is depicted in Fig. 2.8, while the cau-

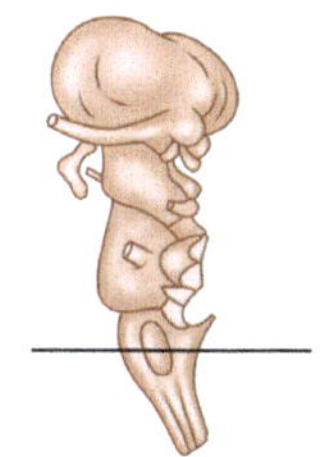

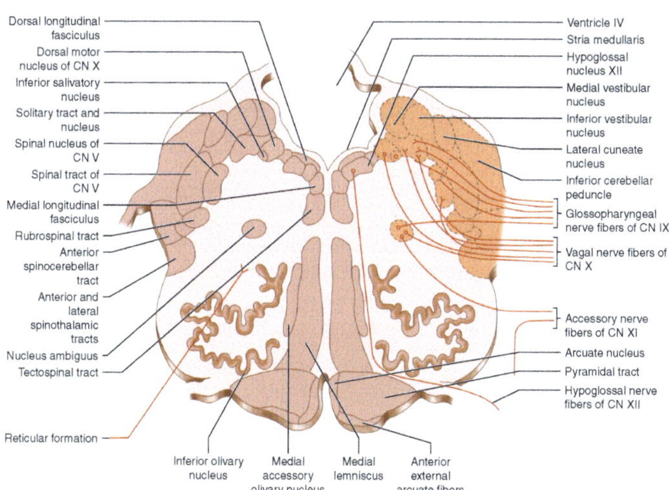

Fig. 2.8 Transverse section through the mid-medulla at the level of the inferior olivary nucleus (indicated by a locator diagram), showing the olivary complex, hypoglossal and dorsal vagal nuclei, solitary nucleus, vestibular nuclei, inferior cerebellar peduncle, cranial nerve root fibers (CN IX, X, XI, XII), and the major ascending and descending tracts

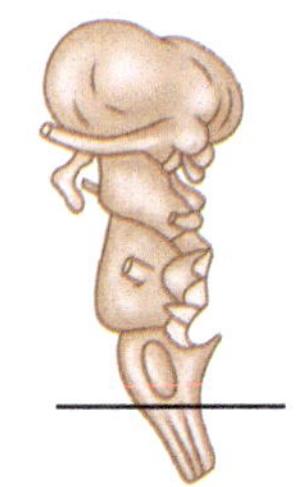

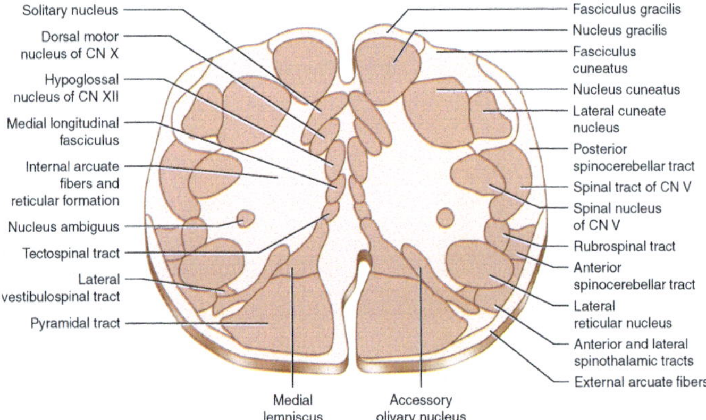

Fig. 2.9 Transverse section through the caudal medulla at the level just below the inferior olivary nucleus (indicated by a locator diagram), showing the posterior column nuclei, spinocerebellar and spinothalamic tracts, spinal trigeminal nucleus and tract, hypoglossal and dorsal vagal nuclei, solitary nucleus, nucleus ambiguus, medial lemniscus, and pyramidal tract

dal medulla is depicted in Fig. 2.9. Figure 2.10 depicts the cervicomedullary junction. Figure 2.11 shows detailed depictions of the cervicomedullary junction.

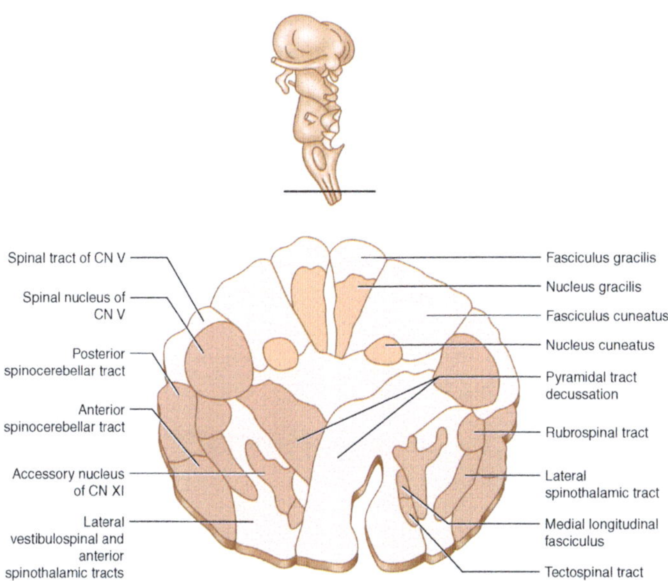

Fig. 2.10 Transverse section through the cervicomedullary junction at the level of the pyramidal decussation (indicated by a locator diagram of the brainstem), showing the major tracts and nuclei including the posterior column fasciculi and their nuclei, spinocerebellar tracts, spinothalamic tracts, corticospinal fibers, and spinal nucleus and tract of CN V

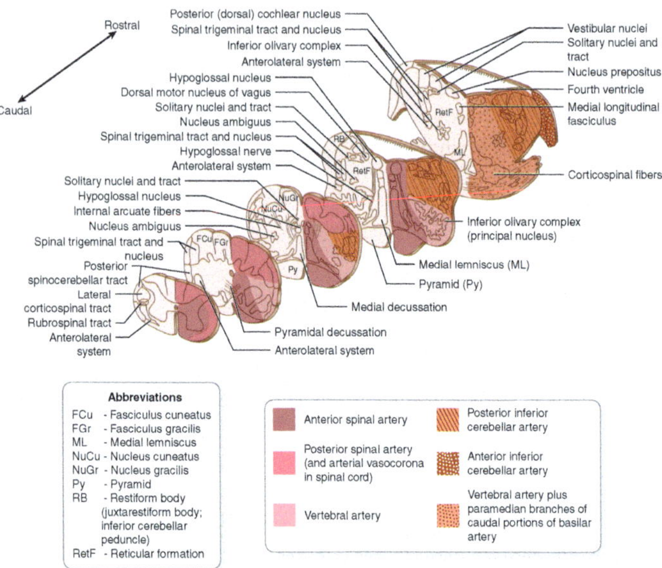

Fig. 2.11 Three-dimensional reconstruction of sequential transverse sections through the caudal medulla and cervicomedullary junction (caudal to rostral), depicting the major tracts and nuclei at each level, with an accompanying legend of abbreviations and color-coded arterial territories (anterior spinal, posterior spinal, vertebral, PICA, and AICA)

Critical Functional Centers of the Medulla

Cardiovascular Centers

The medulla contains the cardiovascular control center, which includes distinct regions for vasomotor regulation and cardiac control. The vasomotor center, located in the rostral ventrolateral medulla, regulates blood pressure through control of sympathetic outflow to blood vessels. The cardiac center modulates heart rate and contractility through both sympathetic and parasympathetic (vagal) pathways. These centers integrate input from baroreceptors, chemoreceptors, and higher brain regions to maintain cardiovascular homeostasis.

Medullary Respiratory Centers

The medulla houses the primary respiratory rhythm generator in the ventral respiratory group and the dorsal respiratory group. The pre-Bötzinger complex, located in the ventrolateral medulla, is believed to be the primary pacemaker for respiratory rhythm generation. These centers generate the basic respiratory rhythm and pattern, which is then modulated by input from the pontine respiratory centers, chemoreceptors (monitoring CO_2, O_2, and pH), and mechanoreceptors in the lungs. Damage to the medullary respiratory centers can be fatal, as these regions are essential for spontaneous breathing.

Additional Autonomic Centers

The medulla also contains centers for vomiting (area postrema and nucleus tractus solitarius), swallowing, coughing, sneezing, and hiccupping. These reflexes are coordinated by neurons in the reticular formation and specific cranial nerve nuclei.

Major Anatomical Structures of the Medulla

Pyramids

The pyramids are prominent paired longitudinal elevations on the anterior surface of the medulla. Each pyramid contains approximately one million corticospinal fibers originating from the motor cortex. At the caudal end of the medulla, approximately 75–90% of these fibers decussate (cross to the opposite side) at the pyramidal decussation to form the lateral corticospinal tract. This anatomical crossing explains the contralateral control of voluntary movement—the left motor cortex controls the right side of the body and vice versa. The remaining 10–25% of fibers continue ipsilaterally as the anterior (ventral) corticospinal tract.

Inferior Olivary Nuclear Complex

The inferior olivary nuclei are large, convoluted nuclei located laterally in the medulla, creating visible elevations called the olives on the anterolateral medullary surface. These nuclei receive input from multiple sources including the cerebral cortex, red nucleus (via rubroolivary fibers in the central tegmental tract), and spinal cord. The inferior olivary nuclei project climbing fibers to the cerebellar cortex via the inferior cerebellar peduncle, playing a crucial role in motor learning, timing, and coordination. Each inferior olive contains approximately 500,000 neurons.

Dorsal Column Nuclei

The dorsal columns of the spinal cord (fasciculus gracilis and fasciculus cuneatus) carry fine touch, vibration, and proprioceptive information from the body. These first-order sensory neurons terminate in the nucleus gracilis (lower body) and nucleus cuneatus (upper body) in the caudal medulla. Second-order neurons from these nuclei decussate as internal arcuate fibers to form the medial lemniscus, which ascends to the ventral posterolateral (VPL) nucleus of the thalamus. The somatotopic organization is preserved, with lower limb representation ventral and upper limb representation dorsal.

Cerebellar Peduncles

The inferior cerebellar peduncles (restiform bodies) connect the medulla to the cerebellum. These peduncles carry multiple afferent pathways to the cerebellum, including:

- Climbing fibers from the contralateral inferior olivary nucleus.
- Dorsal spinocerebellar tract (unconscious proprioception from lower body).
- Cuneocerebellar tract (unconscious proprioception from upper body).
- Vestibulocerebellar fibers from the vestibular nuclei and directly from CN VIII.
- Reticulocerebellar fibers.

Cranial Nerves Originating from the Medulla

The medulla gives rise to four cranial nerves that control various motor, sensory, and autonomic functions:

Glossopharyngeal Nerve (Cranial Nerve IX)
CN IX provides motor innervation to the stylopharyngeus muscle, carries taste and general sensation from the posterior third of the tongue, provides sensation to the pharynx and middle ear, and carries parasympathetic fibers to the parotid gland. The nucleus ambiguus provides the motor component, the nucleus tractus solitarius receives taste input, and the inferior salivatory nucleus provides the parasympathetic component.

Vagus Nerve (Cranial Nerve X)
CN X is the most widely distributed cranial nerve, with extensive autonomic innervation to thoracic and abdominal organs. It provides motor innervation to muscles of the palate, pharynx, and larynx; carries taste from the epiglottis; provides sensation to the external ear; and supplies parasympathetic innervation to the heart, lungs, and digestive tract down to the splenic flexure. The dorsal motor nucleus of the vagus provides parasympathetic output, the nucleus ambiguus provides motor fibers, and the nucleus tractus solitarius receives visceral sensory input.

Accessory Nerve (Cranial Nerve XI)
CN XI has both cranial and spinal roots. The cranial portion (internal branch) joins the vagus nerve to innervate laryngeal muscles. The spinal portion (external branch) arises from the upper cervical spinal cord (C1–C5) and innervates the sternocleidomastoid and trapezius muscles, controlling head movement and shoulder elevation.

Hypoglossal Nerve (Cranial Nerve XII)
CN XII innervates all intrinsic and most extrinsic muscles of the tongue, controlling tongue movement during speech, swallowing, and mastication. The hypoglossal nucleus is located in the dorso-

medial medulla beneath the hypoglossal trigone in the floor of the fourth ventricle. Unilateral hypoglossal nerve lesions cause the tongue to deviate toward the side of the lesion due to unopposed action of the contralateral genioglossus muscle.

Distinctive Neurochemical Nuclei of the Brainstem

The brainstem contains several important nuclei defined by their neurotransmitter phenotype. These neurochemically distinct cell groups have widespread projections throughout the central nervous system and modulate diverse functions including arousal, mood, motivation, motor control, and autonomic regulation.

Dopaminergic Systems

Substantia Nigra Pars Compacta (A9)

As discussed earlier, the substantia nigra pars compacta contains dopaminergic neurons that project to all regions of the striatum via the nigrostriatal pathway. This pathway is critical for the initiation and smooth execution of voluntary movements. These neurons show early and severe degeneration in Parkinson's disease, resulting in the characteristic motor symptoms. When approximately 60–70% of substantia nigra dopaminergic neurons are lost, parkinsonian symptoms become clinically apparent.

Ventral Tegmental Area (A10)

The ventral tegmental area (VTA) is located medial to the substantia nigra in the midbrain tegmentum. VTA dopaminergic neurons project extensively throughout the brain, including the ventral striatum (nucleus accumbens), prefrontal cortex, cingulate cortex, amygdala, thalamus, and hypothalamus. These projections form several important pathways: the mesolimbic pathway (to the nucleus accumbens and limbic structures), involved in reward, motivation, and emotion; and the mesocortical pathway (to the frontal and temporal cortex), involved in cognition, working memory, and executive function. The VTA dopaminergic system is implicated in addiction, reward processing, and psychiatric disorders including schizophrenia. VTA neurons show relatively late degeneration in Parkinson's disease compared to substantia nigra neurons, which may explain the preservation of some cognitive and motivational functions early in the disease course.

Dopamine Receptors

Dopamine acts through two main receptor families with opposing effects on intracellular signaling. D1 receptors couple to Gs proteins and increase intracellular cyclic AMP (cAMP) levels, generally having excitatory effects. D2 receptors couple to Gi proteins and decrease intracellular cAMP levels, generally having inhibitory effects. The balance between D1 and D2 receptor activation is crucial for normal basal ganglia function and movement control.

Median Eminence

A third important dopaminergic system involves neurons in the hypothalamic arcuate nucleus that release dopamine into the hypothalamic-hypophyseal portal system at the median eminence. This dopamine (also called prolactin-inhibiting hormone) travels to the anterior pituitary where it inhibits prolactin secretion by lactotroph cells. Disruption of this pathway (e.g., by pituitary tumors or certain medications) can result in hyperprolactinemia.

Noradrenergic System

The locus coeruleus (described earlier under the pons section) represents the major noradrenergic nucleus of the brainstem. The nucleus subceruleus, located ventral to the locus coeruleus, also contains noradrenergic neurons. These systems project widely throughout the CNS and play crucial roles in arousal, attention, stress response, and autonomic regulation.

Serotonergic System

Raphe Nuclei

The raphe nuclei are a series of serotonergic cell groups distributed throughout the midline of the brainstem, spanning the midbrain (mesencephalic raphe), pons (pontine raphe), and medulla (medullary raphe). Despite being located in the midline, these nuclei project extensively and diffusely throughout the entire central nervous system, including all regions of the cerebral cortex, limbic system, basal ganglia, thalamus, hypothalamus, cerebellum, and spinal cord. The raphe nuclei play crucial roles in regulating the level of arousal, modulating pain transmission, regulating mood and emotion, and controlling the sleep-wake cycle. Serotonin from the raphe nuclei is particularly important in REM sleep regulation. The raphe nuclei are major targets of selective serotonin reuptake inhibitors (SSRIs) and other antidepressant medications. These projections are carried in part through the medial forebrain bundle.

Cholinergic Systems

Several important cholinergic nuclei are located in the basal forebrain region, though technically not in the brainstem proper, their connections with brainstem structures merit discussion:

Medial Septal Nucleus (Ch1)

Located anterosuperiorly in the basal forebrain, this cholinergic nucleus projects to the hippocampus via the fornix (important for memory formation) and to the habenula and ventral tegmental area via the stria medullaris.

Vertical and Horizontal Limbs of the Diagonal Band of Broca (Ch2 and Ch3)

These nuclei send cholinergic projections to the hippocampus (via fornix), habenula and VTA (via stria medullaris), and the olfactory bulb (particularly from Ch3). These connections are important for memory, emotion, and olfactory processing.

Nucleus Basalis of Meynert (Ch4)

Located posteroinferiorly in the substantia innominata, ventral to the anterior commissure and globus pallidus, the nucleus basalis contains large cholinergic neurons that project extensively to the cerebral cortex and amygdala. These projections may regulate the sleep-wake cycle, attention, and cortical processing. The nucleus basalis shows early pathological changes in both Parkinson's disease (accumulation of Lewy bodies) and Alzheimer's disease (neuronal degeneration), contributing to the cognitive impairments seen in these conditions. The projections travel through multiple pathways including the fornix, cingulum bundle, and external capsule.

Histaminergic System

Tuberomammillary Nucleus

Located in the posterior hypothalamus, the tuberomammillary nucleus contains histaminergic neurons that project to widespread areas including the cerebral cortex, hippocampus, amygdala, olfactory bulb, striatum, pallidum, hypothalamus, and most cranial nerve nuclei and reticular formation. Histaminergic projections play important roles in regulating arousal and attention, the sleep-wake cycle, and feeding behavior. Histamine acts through three main receptor types: H1 receptors (found in gastric mucosa), H2 receptors (mediating peripheral effects), and H3 receptors (mediating central nervous system effects). First-generation antihistamines that cross the blood-brain barrier and block H1 receptors cause sedation, while newer antihistamines that do not readily cross into the CNS cause less drowsiness.

Major Brainstem Tracts

Medial Longitudinal Fasciculus (MLF)

The MLF is a heavily myelinated fiber bundle that extends from the upper midbrain to the cervical spinal cord, located close to the midline in the dorsal tegmentum. It coordinates eye movements with head movements and postural adjustments by connecting the vestibular nuclei with the oculomotor, trochlear, and abducens nuclei. The MLF carries several types of fibers: vestibular fibers from the medial and superior vestibular nuclei project bilaterally to the abducens nuclei, contralaterally to the trochlear nuclei, and contralaterally to the oculomotor nuclei. Fibers from the medial vestibular nucleus also project contralaterally to the interstitial nucleus of Cajal (INC), which is involved in vertical gaze movement, while fibers from the superior vestibular nucleus project ipsilaterally to the INC. Additionally, the MLF contains abducens interneurons that connect each abducens nucleus to the contralateral medial rectus subnucleus of the oculomotor nucleus, enabling coordinated horizontal conjugate gaze. Lesions of the MLF result in internuclear ophthalmoplegia, characterized by impaired adduction of the eye on the side of the lesion and nystagmus of the abducting eye.

Central Tegmental Tract

This tract represents a major pathway for fibers traversing the brainstem. Its primary component is the descending rubroolivary tract, which carries fibers from the ipsilateral red nucleus to the inferior olivary nuclear complex. These connections are important for motor learning and coordination. The central tegmental tract also serves as the major route by which reticular formation fibers ascend to the thalamus, contributing to arousal and consciousness.

Posterior (Dorsal) Longitudinal Fasciculus

This bidirectional fiber bundle connects the hypothalamus with the brainstem reticular formation, allowing integration of autonomic and behavioral responses with brainstem reflexes and visceral functions.

Medial Lemniscus

The medial lemniscus carries secondary sensory fibers from the dorsal column nuclei (gracile and cuneate nuclei) to the ventral posterolateral (VPL) nucleus of the thalamus. These fibers convey fine touch, vibration sense, and proprioception from the body. The tract maintains a somatotopic organization throughout its course, with the lower limb represented ventrally and the upper limb represented dorsally. After decussating as internal arcuate fibers in the medulla, the medial lemniscus ascends through the brainstem, gradually rotating from a vertical to a horizontal orientation as it approaches the thalamus.

Lateral Lemniscus

The lateral lemniscus is a major component of the ascending auditory pathway. It transmits sound information from the cochlear nuclei and superior olivary complex to the inferior colliculus and eventually to the auditory cortex. This pathway plays an important role in sound localization and auditory processing. The lateral lemniscus contains tonotopically organized fibers that preserve the frequency information encoded in the cochlea.

Trigeminothalamic Tracts

The trigeminal sensory system projects to the thalamus via two main pathways. The dorsal (posterior) trigeminothalamic tract carries discriminative touch information from the principal sensory nucleus, while the ventral (anterior) trigeminothalamic tract carries pain and temperature information from the spinal trigeminal nucleus. Both pathways decussate and project to the ventral posteromedial (VPM) nucleus of the thalamus.

Medial Forebrain Bundle

This is a complex bundle of ascending and descending fibers connecting the brainstem with the forebrain, particularly the hypothalamus, septal area, and nucleus accumbens. It carries projections from multiple neurochemical systems including dopaminergic fibers from the VTA to the nucleus accumbens (mesolimbic pathway), serotonergic fibers from the raphe nuclei, and connections from the interpeduncular nucleus to the hypothalamus.

Brainstem Arterial Supply

Understanding the vascular supply to the brainstem is clinically crucial, as brainstem strokes can produce characteristic syndromes depending on which vessels are affected. The brainstem receives its blood supply from the vertebrobasilar system through a consistent pattern of three types of arterial branches: paramedian perforators, short circumferential penetrators, and long circumferential penetrators.

Midbrain Vascular Supply

The midbrain receives blood supply anteriorly from the posterior cerebral artery (PCA) and posteriorly from the superior cerebellar artery (SCA) and the quadrigeminal artery (a branch of the PCA). Paramedian branches supply the medial structures including the oculomotor nucleus, red nucleus, and medial cerebral peduncle. Circumferential branches supply the tectum, substantia nigra, and lateral portions of the tegmentum.

Pontine Vascular Supply

The pons is supplied primarily by branches arising directly from the basilar artery. Paramedian perforating arteries supply the medial basis pontis and portions of the tegmentum, including the medial lemniscus and paramedian pontine reticular formation. Short circumferential penetrating arteries supply lateral tegmental structures. Long circumferential arteries, particularly the anterior inferior cerebellar artery (AICA) and superior cerebellar artery, supply more lateral and dorsal pontine structures and the cerebellar peduncles.

Medullary Vascular Supply

The medulla receives blood from three main sources. Paramedian perforators arise from the anterior spinal artery (which is formed by the union of branches from both vertebral arteries) and supply the pyramids, medial lemniscus, and hypoglossal nucleus. Short circumferential penetrators arise directly from the vertebral arteries and supply the inferior olivary nuclei. Long circumferential penetrators, primarily from the posterior inferior cerebellar artery (PICA), supply the lateral medulla including the vestibular nuclei, nucleus ambiguus, descending sympathetic fibers, spinothalamic tract, and inferior cerebellar peduncle. The posterior spinal arteries, which branch from PICA, supply the most posterior portions of the caudal medulla including the dorsal column nuclei.

Occlusion of PICA results in lateral medullary syndrome (Wallenberg syndrome), one of the most common brainstem stroke syndromes, characterized by vertigo, ataxia, dysphagia, ipsilateral Horner syndrome, loss of pain and temperature sensation on the ipsilateral face and contralateral body, and other signs depending on the extent of infarction.

Clinical Significance and Summary

The brainstem, despite its relatively small size, is one of the most critical regions of the central nervous system. Its importance is reflected in several key functional domains:

Motor Control and Coordination

Major descending motor pathways, including the corticospinal and corticobulbar tracts, traverse the brainstem. The brainstem houses important motor nuclei including the red nucleus, substantia nigra, and cranial nerve motor nuclei that control eye movements, facial expression, mastication, swallowing, and phonation. Cerebellar connections through the three peduncle pairs allow integration of motor commands with balance and coordination. Damage to brainstem motor pathways or nuclei can result in weakness, paralysis, dysarthria, dysphagia, or movement disorders.

Sensory Processing and Relay

Ascending sensory pathways carrying touch, pain, temperature, proprioception, auditory information, and vestibular information all pass through or synapse in the brainstem. The brainstem contains important relay nuclei including the dorsal column nuclei, trigeminal sensory nuclei, cochlear nuclei, vestibular nuclei, and inferior olivary nuclei. Processing of sensory information begins in the brainstem before relay to the thalamus and cortex. Brainstem lesions can cause sensory loss, pain, numbness, hearing loss, or balance disturbances.

Autonomic and Vital Functions

The brainstem, particularly the medulla, contains vital centers that regulate cardiovascular function (heart rate and blood pressure), respiratory rhythm and pattern, and various protective reflexes (cough, gag, vomiting). These functions are essential for survival, and damage to these centers can be rapidly fatal. The concept of "brain death" in clinical practice largely relates to irreversible loss of brainstem function.

Consciousness and Arousal

The reticular formation and its ascending projections (the reticular activating system) are essential for maintaining consciousness and arousal. The widespread projections from neurochemically distinct nuclei (locus coeruleus, raphe nuclei, ventral tegmental area) modulate cortical excitability, attention, and the sleep-wake cycle. Brainstem lesions affecting these systems can result in altered consciousness, coma, or disorders of sleep and wakefulness.

Cranial Nerve Functions

Ten of the twelve cranial nerves (CN III–XII) originate from the brainstem, providing motor, sensory, and autonomic innervation to structures of the head and neck. These nerves control eye movements, facial sensation and movement, hearing and balance, taste, swallowing, phonation, and tongue movement. Brainstem lesions often affect multiple cranial nerves simultaneously, producing characteristic clinical syndromes that help localize the lesion.

Understanding brainstem anatomy is fundamental for clinical neuroscience and neurological practice. The compact organization of the brainstem, with multiple critical structures in close proximity, means that even small lesions can produce complex and devastating neurological syndromes. Careful neurological examination, combined with knowledge of brainstem anatomy, allows clinicians to localize lesions with remarkable precision and guide appropriate diagnostic and therapeutic interventions. The brainstem truly represents the vital core of the nervous system, integrating sensory and motor information, maintaining consciousness and vital functions, and serving as the essential link between the brain and the rest of the body.

The Cranial Nerves

3

Introduction

The cranial nerves represent one of the most clinically significant and anatomically complex components of the nervous system. Unlike the spinal nerves, which emerge segmentally from the spinal cord with relatively uniform organization, the 12 pairs of cranial nerves emerge directly from various levels of the brain and exhibit remarkable diversity in their structure, function, and distribution. Numbered I through XII using Roman numerals in rostral-to-caudal sequence, these nerves serve a vast array of functions that are essential for human sensory perception, motor control, and autonomic regulation.

The cranial nerves can be broadly categorized based on their functional roles. Several nerves are purely sensory, including the olfactory nerve (CN I) for smell, the optic nerve (CN II) for vision, and the vestibulocochlear nerve (CN VIII) for hearing and balance. Others are purely motor, such as the oculomotor (CN III), trochlear (CN IV), abducens (CN VI), accessory (CN XI), and hypoglossal (CN XII) nerves, which control eye movements, shoulder elevation, and tongue movements, respectively. However, many cranial nerves are mixed, carrying both sensory and motor fibers, and several also carry parasympathetic autonomic fibers. These mixed nerves—including the trigeminal (CN V), facial (CN VII), glossopharyngeal (CN IX), and vagus (CN X)—exhibit

V. Yanamadala, *Essential Neuroanatomy*,
https://doi.org/10.1007/978-3-032-26877-8_3

the most complex anatomical organization and clinical significance.

Understanding cranial nerve anatomy requires familiarity with the classical functional component system, which categorizes nerve fibers based on their functional and developmental origins. This system recognizes seven types of functional components:

- *General somatic afferent (GSA)*: Sensory fibers carrying general sensation (pain, temperature, touch, pressure, proprioception) from skin and mucous membranes.
- *General visceral afferent (GVA)*: Sensory fibers carrying visceral sensation from internal organs, blood vessels, and glands.
- *Special visceral afferent (SVA)*: Special sensory fibers for taste and smell, which develop from the visceral arches.
- *Special somatic afferent (SSA)*: Special sensory fibers for vision, hearing, and equilibrium.
- *General somatic efferent (GSE)*: Motor fibers to muscles derived from somites (including extraocular and tongue muscles).
- *General visceral efferent (GVE)*: Parasympathetic preganglionic motor fibers to smooth muscle, cardiac muscle, and glands.
- *Special visceral efferent (SVE)*: Motor fibers to muscles derived from the branchial (pharyngeal) arches, including muscles of mastication, facial expression, pharynx, larynx, and upper esophagus.

This functional component classification provides a systematic framework for understanding the diverse roles of cranial nerves and helps predict the clinical consequences of nerve injury. For instance, damage to a nerve carrying SVE fibers will affect muscles of branchial arch origin, while injury to GVE fibers will disrupt parasympathetic autonomic function. These are schematically represented in Fig. 3.1.

The cranial nerve examination represents an essential component of the neurological examination, providing critical information for lesion localization and differential diagnosis. A thorough

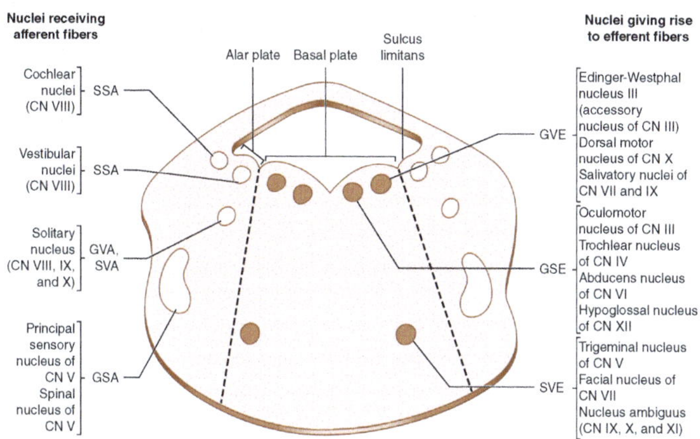

Fig. 3.1 Schematic cross section of the brainstem illustrating the functional organization of cranial nerve nuclei within the alar and basal plates, separated by the sulcus limitans, with classification into GSA, SSA, GVA/SVA, GVE, GSE, and SVE functional columns and their associated cranial nerve nuclei

understanding of cranial nerve anatomy, including the locations of cranial nerve nuclei within the brainstem, the course of nerve fibers through the skull base, and the peripheral distribution of nerve branches, enables clinicians to distinguish between peripheral nerve lesions, brainstem nuclear lesions, and supranuclear (upper motor neuron) lesions. This distinction has profound implications for diagnosis, prognosis, and treatment planning.

Systematic Overview of the Cranial Nerves

The following section provides a comprehensive overview of each cranial nerve, proceeding in numerical order from CN I through CN XII. For each nerve, we will discuss its functional classification, origin within the central nervous system, anatomical pathway, major branches when applicable, and primary clinical correlations. This systematic approach establishes the foundation for the more detailed anatomical discussions that follow in subsequent sections.

Cranial Nerve I: Olfactory Nerve

Functional Classification: Special Sensory (SSA/SVA)—Olfaction.

Origin and pathway: The olfactory system is unique among cranial nerves in that it is the only sensory system with a direct projection to the cerebral cortex without an obligatory thalamic relay. Olfactory receptor neurons are bipolar neurons located in the olfactory epithelium in the roof of the nasal cavity, superior nasal conchae, and upper portion of the nasal septum. These specialized neurons are continuously regenerated from basal cells throughout life, making them unique among neurons in their regenerative capacity.

Each olfactory receptor neuron extends a single dendrite to the epithelial surface, where it expands into an olfactory knob bearing multiple cilia that contain the odorant receptors. The unmyelinated axons of these neurons, collectively referred to as olfactory fila, pass through the cribriform plate of the ethmoid bone in small bundles to enter the anterior cranial fossa. These approximately 20 bundles on each side constitute the olfactory nerves proper. The olfactory fila synapse with second-order neurons in the olfactory bulb, forming complex synaptic structures called glomeruli.

Within the olfactory bulb, mitral cells and tufted cells receive input from olfactory receptor neurons. These second-order neurons send their axons posteriorly through the olfactory tract to reach the primary olfactory cortex. The olfactory tract divides into medial and lateral olfactory striae at the olfactory trigone. The lateral stria carries most fibers to the primary olfactory cortex, which includes the piriform cortex (located in the anterior temporal lobe), periamygdaloid cortex, and portions of the entorhinal cortex. The medial stria contains fibers that cross to the contralateral olfactory bulb via the anterior commissure.

From the primary olfactory cortex, projections extend to the orbitofrontal cortex (conscious perception and discrimination of odors), amygdala (emotional responses to odors), hippocampus (olfactory memory), and hypothalamus (autonomic responses to odors). This direct connection between the olfactory system and the limbic system explains the powerful ability of odors to evoke memories and emotions.

Clinical relevance: Anosmia (complete loss of smell) or hyposmia (reduced sense of smell) can result from multiple etiologies. Head trauma, particularly frontal impact, can shear the delicate olfactory fila as they pass through the cribriform plate, resulting in permanent anosmia. Upper respiratory infections, both viral and bacterial, can damage the olfactory epithelium and cause temporary or permanent olfactory dysfunction. Chronic rhinosinusitis and nasal polyps can mechanically obstruct airflow to the olfactory epithelium. Importantly, olfactory dysfunction is increasingly recognized as an early marker of neurodegenerative diseases, particularly Alzheimer's disease and Parkinson's disease, often preceding motor or cognitive symptoms by years. Olfactory groove meningiomas and other tumors at the base of the frontal lobe can compress the olfactory bulbs and tracts. Parosmia (distorted smell perception) and phantosmia (perception of odors without external stimuli) can occur with partial olfactory nerve injury or during recovery. Congenital anosmia may occur in Kallmann syndrome, associated with hypogonadotropic hypogonadism due to failure of migration of GnRH neurons and olfactory bulb development.

Cranial Nerve II: Optic Nerve

Functional Classification: Special Sensory (SSA)—Vision.

Embryological significance: The optic nerve is technically not a true peripheral nerve but rather an extension of the central nervous system. During embryological development, the retina forms as an outgrowth (evagination) of the diencephalon, and the optic nerve represents a central nervous system white matter tract. Consequently, the optic nerve is ensheathed by all three meningeal layers (dura, arachnoid, and pia mater) and is surrounded by cerebrospinal fluid in the subarachnoid space. This anatomical relationship explains why increased intracranial pressure can cause papilledema (optic disc swelling).

Retinal organization: The neural retina consists of multiple layers of neurons that process visual information before transmitting it to the brain. Photoreceptors (rods for scotopic/night vision and cones for photopic/day vision and color vision) transduce light into electrical signals. These signals are processed through a complex network of bipolar cells, horizontal cells, and amacrine cells before reaching retinal ganglion cells. The axons of retinal ganglion cells converge at the optic disc (also called the optic nerve head or papilla), where they turn posteriorly to form the optic nerve. The optic disc contains no photoreceptors, creating the physiological blind spot in each eye's visual field.

Course of the optic nerve: The optic nerve exits the posterior aspect of the globe and travels through the orbital fat within the muscle cone formed by the extraocular muscles. The intraorbital segment of the optic nerve measures approximately 25–30 mm in length and follows a slightly S-shaped course, allowing for eye movement without placing traction on the nerve. The central retinal artery and vein enter the optic nerve approximately 10–15 mm posterior to the globe and travel within the center of the nerve.

The nerve exits the orbit through the optic canal (optic foramen), a bony channel in the lesser wing of the sphenoid bone that also transmits the ophthalmic artery. The intracanalicular segment measures approximately 6–10 mm. After exiting the optic canal, the nerve enters the middle cranial fossa and runs posteromedially for 10–16 mm before reaching the optic chiasm.

Optic chiasm and decussation: At the optic chiasm, located superior to the pituitary gland and anterior to the pituitary stalk, a partial decussation of optic nerve fibers occurs based on retinotopic organization. Fibers from the nasal hemiretina (which receive light from the temporal visual field) decussate to the contralateral side, while fibers from the temporal hemiretina (which receive light from the nasal visual field) remain ipsilateral. This arrangement ensures that each optic tract carries information from the contralateral visual field. Fibers from the inferior nasal retina loop anteriorly into the contralateral optic nerve before joining the optic tract, forming Wilbrand's knee—a clinically significant anatomical detail explaining certain visual field defect patterns.

Optic tract and central visual pathways: After the chiasm, the reorganized fibers continue as the optic tracts, which sweep around the cerebral peduncles to reach the lateral geniculate nucleus (LGN) of the thalamus. The LGN is a six-layered structure that maintains retinotopic organization, with layers 1, 4, and 6 receiving input from the contralateral eye and layers 2, 3, and 5 from the ipsilateral eye. Magnocellular layers (1 and 2) process motion and coarse spatial information, while parvocellular layers (3–6) process fine detail and color information.

From the LGN, third-order neurons project through the optic radiations (geniculocalcarine tract) to the primary visual cortex (V1, Brodmann area 17) in the occipital lobe. The optic radiations have two main components: fibers representing the superior visual field travel through the temporal lobe (Meyer's loop) before reaching the inferior bank of the calcarine sulcus, while fibers representing the inferior visual field travel through the parietal lobe to reach the superior bank of the calcarine sulcus. The macula, which serves central vision, has a disproportionately large representation in the posterior occipital cortex.

Clinical relevance: The anatomical organization of the visual pathway allows precise lesion localization based on visual field defects. Complete optic nerve lesions cause ipsilateral monocular blindness with loss of both direct and consensual pupillary light reflexes when light is shone in the affected eye (afferent pupillary defect or Marcus Gunn pupil). Lesions at the optic chiasm, most commonly from pituitary adenomas or craniopharyngiomas, cause bitemporal hemianopia due to damage to crossing nasal retinal fibers. Optic tract lesions cause contralateral homonymous hemianopia with preserved central vision initially. Lesions of Meyer's loop in the temporal lobe cause contralateral superior quadrantanopia ("pie in the sky" defect). Complete lesions of the optic radiations or visual cortex cause contralateral homonymous hemianopia, often with macular sparing due to dual blood supply to the occipital pole from both posterior cerebral and middle cerebral arteries. Optic neuritis, commonly associated with multiple sclerosis, presents with painful vision loss, decreased color perception, and a central scotoma. Papilledema from increased intracranial pressure initially causes enlargement of the blind spot without affecting visual acuity. Glaucoma causes characteristic optic nerve cupping and progressive peripheral visual field loss due to damage to ganglion cell axons at the optic nerve head.

Cranial Nerve III: Oculomotor Nerve

Functional Classification: Motor—GSE (Somatic Motor) and GVE (Parasympathetic).

Nuclear organization: The oculomotor nuclear complex is located in the midbrain tegmentum at the level of the superior colliculus, ventral to the periaqueductal gray matter and medial to the medial longitudinal fasciculus. This complex consists of multiple subnuclei, each innervating specific extraocular muscles with precise topographic organization:

- The dorsal nucleus (also called the caudal central nucleus or nucleus of Perlia) is a midline unpaired structure that may be involved in convergence, though its precise function remains debated.
- The central caudal nucleus is also unpaired and innervates both levator palpebrae superioris muscles bilaterally, explaining why ptosis from a nuclear lesion is typically bilateral.
- Paired lateral subnuclei innervate the inferior rectus, medial rectus, and inferior oblique muscles ipsilaterally.
- A paired dorsomedial subnucleus innervates the superior rectus muscle, but the fibers decussate before exiting the brainstem, so each superior rectus is innervated by the contralateral oculomotor nucleus.

The Edinger-Westphal nucleus (accessory oculomotor nucleus) is located dorsal to the main motor nucleus and contains preganglionic parasympathetic neurons that provide autonomic innervation to the eye. These fibers ultimately control pupillary constriction and accommodation.

Course and distribution: Oculomotor nerve fibers exit the brainstem ventrally through the interpeduncular fossa (between the cerebral peduncles) in the anterior midbrain. The nerve passes forward between the posterior cerebral artery superiorly and the superior cerebellar artery inferiorly, a region where aneurysms commonly develop and can compress the nerve. The oculomotor nerve then travels anteriorly in the lateral wall of the cavernous sinus, positioned superior to the trochlear nerve. The parasympathetic fibers travel superficially within the nerve, making them vulnerable to external compression.

The nerve enters the orbit through the superior orbital fissure within the annulus of Zinn (common tendinous ring) and divides into superior and inferior divisions:

- *Superior division*: Innervates the superior rectus muscle (elevates eye, particularly in abduction) and the levator palpebrae superioris muscle (elevates upper eyelid).
- *Inferior division*: Innervates the medial rectus (adducts eye), inferior rectus (depresses eye, particularly in adduction), and inferior oblique (elevates eye in adduction and extorts). The inferior division also carries preganglionic parasympathetic fibers that synapse in the ciliary ganglion.

Parasympathetic pathway: Preganglionic parasympathetic fibers from the Edinger-Westphal nucleus travel via the branch to the inferior oblique to reach the ciliary ganglion, located in the posterior orbit lateral to the optic nerve. In the ciliary ganglion, these preganglionic fibers synapse with postganglionic neurons. Short ciliary nerves (usually 6–10 in number) carry postganglionic parasympathetic fibers from the ciliary ganglion to the eye, where they innervate:

- *Sphincter pupillae muscle*: Causes pupillary constriction (miosis) in response to light or accommodation.
- *Ciliary muscle*: Contraction allows the lens to become more spherical (increasing refractive power) for accommodation to near objects.

Clinical relevance: Oculomotor nerve palsy produces a characteristic constellation of findings. Complete third nerve palsy causes ptosis (drooping eyelid from levator palpebrae paralysis), the eye positioned "down and out" (due to unopposed action of the lateral rectus [CN VI] and superior oblique [CN IV]), restricted adduction and elevation, diplopia, and mydriasis (dilated pupil) when parasympathetic fibers are involved. The distinction between "pupil-sparing" and "pupil-involving" third nerve palsies has important diagnostic implications. Pupil-sparing palsies suggest microvascular ischemia (common in diabetes mellitus and hypertension), where the vasa nervorum supplying the core of the nerve are affected while the superficial parasympathetic fibers remain functional. In contrast, pupil-involving palsies suggest external compression, most urgently from a posterior communicating artery aneurysm, which compresses the superficial parasympathetic fibers first. This distinction makes a dilated pupil in the context of third nerve palsy a medical emergency requiring urgent neuroimaging. Other causes of third nerve palsy include cavernous sinus lesions, orbital apex lesions, midbrain stroke or hemorrhage, increased intracranial pressure with uncal herniation, inflammatory conditions, and trauma. Nuclear lesions produce distinctive patterns: bilateral ptosis (central caudal nucleus involvement), bilateral superior rectus weakness, or aberrant regeneration. The pupillary light reflex has both an afferent limb (retina → optic nerve → pretectal nuclei) and an efferent limb (Edinger-Westphal nucleus → oculomotor nerve → ciliary ganglion → sphincter pupillae). Testing both direct and consensual light reflexes helps localize lesions.

Cranial Nerve IV: Trochlear Nerve

Functional Classification: Motor—GSE (Somatic Motor to Superior Oblique Muscle).

Nuclear origin and unique anatomical features: The trochlear nucleus is located in the midbrain tegmentum at the level of the inferior colliculus, just caudal to the oculomotor nuclear complex. The trochlear nerve has three unique characteristics that distinguish it from all other cranial nerves: (1) it is the only cranial nerve to exit from the dorsal aspect of the brainstem, (2) it completely decussates before exiting the brainstem (meaning each trochlear nucleus innervates the contralateral superior oblique muscle), and (3) it is the smallest cranial nerve in terms of the number of axons it contains.

Course and distribution: Trochlear nerve fibers exit from the trochlear nucleus and course dorsally and caudally to decussate completely in the superior medullary velum (the roof of the fourth ventricle at the isthmus level) before emerging from the dorsal surface of the brainstem just inferior to the inferior colliculus. The nerve then wraps around the lateral surface of the brainstem in the subarachnoid space, traveling ventrally and rostrally. It has the longest intracranial course of any cranial nerve, making it particularly vulnerable to trauma.

The trochlear nerve passes between the posterior cerebral artery and the superior cerebellar artery before piercing the dura mater to enter the lateral wall of the cavernous sinus, where it runs inferior to the oculomotor nerve. It enters the orbit through the superior orbital fissure, outside the annulus of Zinn (unlike the oculomotor and abducens nerves), and passes medially above the levator palpebrae superioris to reach the superior oblique muscle. The superior oblique muscle originates from the body of the sphenoid bone and its tendon passes through a fibrocartilaginous pulley called the trochlea (from Greek for "pulley") attached to the frontal bone in the superomedial orbit, then turns posterolaterally to insert on the superolateral aspect of the globe behind the equator.

Function of the superior oblique muscle: The superior oblique muscle has three primary actions: (1) depression (downward movement) of the eye, most effective when the eye is adducted; (2) intorsion (internal rotation) of the eye; and (3) abduction. The depressor function is most important clinically. Because the muscle approaches the eye from an anteromedial direction after passing through the trochlea, its actions are complex and depend on the initial position of the eye.

Clinical relevance: Trochlear nerve palsy causes vertical diplopia (double vision with images separated vertically) that characteristically worsens when the patient looks down and toward the nose (down and in), particularly problematic when reading or descending stairs. Patients experience maximum diplopia when attempting to look down with the affected eye adducted, because this is when the superior oblique normally has its greatest depressor action. The unopposed action of the inferior oblique causes relative elevation of the affected eye (hypertropia). Patients typically adopt a compensatory head tilt toward the contralateral shoulder to minimize diplopia by using the intorsion action of the intact superior rectus muscle on the affected side. This head tilt is an important clinical sign. The Parks-Bielschowsky three-step test helps identify which eye and which muscle is affected: Step 1 identifies which eye is higher (hypertrophic), Step 2 determines whether hypertropia worsens in right or left gaze, Step 3 assesses whether hypertropia worsens with head tilt to right or left. Trochlear nerve palsy is most commonly caused by closed head trauma (due to its long intracranial course and dorsal exit making it vulnerable to contrecoup injury), microvascular ischemia (diabetes, hypertension), or congenital anomalies. Bilateral trochlear nerve palsy, though rare, can occur with severe head trauma and causes characteristic alternating hypertropia depending on direction of gaze. Decompensated congenital trochlear palsy may present in adulthood when compensatory mechanisms fail, often evident on review of old photographs showing long-standing head tilt.

Cranial Nerve V: Trigeminal Nerve

Functional Classification: Mixed—GSA (General Somatic Sensory) and SVE (Motor to Muscles of Mastication).

Overview: The trigeminal nerve is the largest cranial nerve and is the principal general sensory nerve of the head and face. It provides somatic sensation from the face, scalp, teeth, oral cavity, nasal cavity, and most of the dura mater. The motor component innervates the muscles of mastication and several other muscles. The nerve's name derives from its three major divisions: ophthalmic (V1), maxillary (V2), and mandibular (V3).

Nuclear organization: The trigeminal nerve has four nuclei in the brainstem:

- *Motor nucleus*: Located in the mid-pons, medial to the main sensory nucleus. Receives bilateral input from the corticobulbar tracts, though the muscles of mastication show predominantly contralateral cortical control.
- *Main (principal or pontine) sensory nucleus*: Located in the mid-pons, processes discriminative touch and conscious proprioception from the face.
- *Spinal trigeminal nucleus*: Extends from the mid-pons through the medulla into the upper cervical spinal cord (C2–C3), divided into three parts: pars oralis (rostral, in pons), pars interpolaris (middle, in medulla), and pars caudalis (caudal, extending to C2). Processes pain and temperature sensation from the face, with a unique somatotopic organization where the mouth is represented rostrally and the peripheral face caudally ("onion skin" distribution).
- *Mesencephalic nucleus*: Located in the midbrain, unique in that it contains the cell bodies of primary sensory neurons (usually located in peripheral ganglia). Carries proprioceptive information from muscles of mastication, extraocular muscles, and teeth.

The trigeminal (gasserian or semilunar) ganglion: The trigeminal ganglion contains the cell bodies of most primary sensory neurons of the trigeminal nerve (except those in the mesencephalic nucleus). It is located in Meckel's cave (cavum trigeminale), a recess of dura mater on the anterior surface of the petrous temporal bone in the middle cranial fossa. The ganglion is crescent-shaped, with the three divisions emerging from its convex anterior border. The motor root of the trigeminal nerve passes beneath the ganglion without synapsing and joins the mandibular division.

Ophthalmic Division (V1)

Distribution: The ophthalmic division is purely sensory and provides sensation to the forehead, upper eyelid, dorsum of the nose, cornea, conjunctiva, anterior scalp, frontal and ethmoid sinuses, and portions of the meninges (particularly the tentorium cerebelli and anterior cranial fossa dura). Before entering the orbit, V1 divides into three main branches:

- *Frontal nerve*: The largest branch. Enters the orbit through the superior orbital fissure outside the annulus of Zinn. Divides into the supraorbital nerve (exits through supraorbital foramen or notch to supply forehead and anterior scalp) and supratrochlear nerve (supplies medial forehead and upper eyelid).
- *Lacrimal nerve*: Enters orbit through superior orbital fissure, runs along lateral orbital wall. Provides sensation to lacrimal gland, lateral upper eyelid, and lateral conjunctiva. Receives secretomotor fibers (for lacrimation) from the pterygopalatine ganglion via a communicating branch from the zygomatic nerve.
- *Nasociliary nerve*: Enters orbit through superior orbital fissure within the annulus of Zinn. Gives off important branches including: the long ciliary nerves (carry sympathetic fibers to dilator pupillae and provide sensation to cornea and iris), anterior and posterior ethmoidal nerves (supply ethmoidal and sphenoidal sinuses), and infratrochlear nerve (supplies medial eyelid, lacrimal sac, and side of nose). The nasociliary nerve also gives off a communicating branch to the ciliary ganglion (sensory root), through which sensory fibers from the eye pass.

Maxillary Division (V2)

Distribution: The maxillary division is purely sensory and provides sensation to the midface, lower eyelid, cheek, side of nose, upper lip, upper teeth and gingiva, hard and soft palate, maxillary sinus, and nasopharynx. V2 exits the skull through the foramen rotundum and enters the pterygopalatine fossa, where it gives off several branches:

- *Zygomatic nerve*: Enters orbit through inferior orbital fissure, divides into zygomaticotemporal (supplies skin over temple) and zygomaticofacial branches (supplies skin over zygoma). Carries secretomotor fibers from pterygopalatine ganglion to lacrimal gland via communication with lacrimal nerve.
- *Pterygopalatine nerves*: Two short nerves connecting to the pterygopalatine ganglion, through which pass: (1) sensory fibers from palate, nasal cavity, and nasopharynx and (2) post-ganglionic parasympathetic fibers from the ganglion to nasal and palatine glands. Branches include greater and lesser palatine nerves (hard and soft palate), nasopalatine nerve (nasal septum and anterior palate), and posterior superior nasal nerves (posterior nasal cavity).
- *Infraorbital nerve*: Continuation of V2 after giving off above branches. Enters orbit through inferior orbital fissure, travels in infraorbital groove and then the canal in floor of orbit, and emerges through infraorbital foramen. Gives off superior alveolar nerves (posterior, middle, anterior) that form superior dental plexus supplying the upper teeth and gingiva. Terminal branches supply the lower eyelid, cheek, side of nose, and upper lip.
- *Meningeal branch*: Supplies the dura mater of middle cranial fossa.

Mandibular Division (V3)

Distribution: The mandibular division is mixed (sensory and motor) and provides sensation to the lower face, lower lip, lower teeth and gingiva, anterior two-thirds of tongue (general sensation, not taste), floor of mouth, chin, temple, external ear, and part of the meninges. It also provides motor innervation to muscles of mastication and several other muscles. V3 exits the skull through the foramen ovale, where it is joined by the motor root of the trigeminal nerve. In the infratemporal fossa, it divides into multiple branches:

Motor branches:

- Nerve to medial pterygoid: Arises from main trunk before division, also gives branches to tensor veli palatini and tensor tympani muscles.
- Masseteric nerve: Crosses mandibular notch to supply masseter muscle.
- Deep temporal nerves (usually anterior and posterior): Supply temporalis muscle.
- Nerve to lateral pterygoid: Supplies lateral pterygoid muscle.
- Mylohyoid nerve: Branch of inferior alveolar nerve, supplies mylohyoid and anterior belly of digastric muscles.

Sensory branches:

- *Meningeal branch (nervus spinosus)*: Re-enters skull through foramen spinosum with middle meningeal artery, supplies dura of middle cranial fossa.
- *Buccal nerve*: Sensory to cheek mucosa and skin over anterior cheek (does NOT innervate buccinator muscle, which is innervated by facial nerve).
- *Auriculotemporal nerve*: Arises by two roots that encircle middle meningeal artery. Carries postganglionic parasympathetic fibers from otic ganglion to parotid gland. Provides sensation to temple, external ear, temporomandibular joint, and parotid region. Important in Frey's syndrome (gustatory sweating after parotid surgery due to aberrant regeneration of parasympathetic fibers to sweat glands).
- *Lingual nerve*: Provides general sensation (touch, pain, temperature, not taste) to anterior two-thirds of tongue, floor of mouth, and lingual gingiva. Joined by chorda tympani branch of facial nerve (carrying taste from anterior two-thirds of tongue and preganglionic parasympathetic fibers to submandibular ganglion). Gives off branches to submandibular ganglion, through which pass parasympathetic fibers to submandibular and sublingual glands.
- *Inferior alveolar nerve*: Enters mandibular foramen on medial aspect of mandibular ramus, travels in mandibular canal giving off branches that form inferior dental plexus supplying lower

teeth and gingiva. Gives off mylohyoid nerve before entering mandible. Terminal branch (mental nerve) emerges through mental foramen to supply chin and lower lip.

Muscles innervated by V3 (motor component):

- *Masseter*: Elevates and protrudes mandible (closes jaw with force).
- *Temporalis*: Elevates and retracts mandible.
- *Medial pterygoid*: Elevates and protrudes mandible, assists in lateral grinding movements.
- *Lateral pterygoid*: Protrudes mandible and produces lateral movements (side to side) for grinding. Bilateral contraction protrudes jaw; unilateral contraction moves jaw to opposite side.
- *Mylohyoid*: Forms floor of mouth, elevates hyoid and tongue during swallowing.
- *Anterior belly of digastric*: Depresses mandible, elevates hyoid.
- *Tensor veli palatini*: Tenses soft palate, opens Eustachian tube during swallowing/yawning.
- *Tensor tympani*: Tenses tympanic membrane, dampens loud sounds.

Clinical relevance: Trigeminal neuralgia (tic douloureux) is characterized by sudden, severe, unilateral, stabbing or electric shock-like pain in the distribution of one or more branches of the trigeminal nerve, most commonly V2 or V3. Episodes last seconds to minutes and are triggered by light tactile stimulation of trigger zones (touching face, chewing, talking, brushing teeth, cold air). Most cases result from vascular compression of the trigeminal nerve root entry zone by an aberrant or ectatic vessel (commonly superior cerebellar artery), causing focal demyelination. Less common causes include multiple sclerosis plaques, posterior fossa tumors, or arteriovenous malformations. Treatment begins with carbamazepine or oxcarbazepine; refractory cases may require microvascular decompression surgery. The corneal reflex tests the integrity of V1 (afferent) and VII (efferent) pathways: touching the cornea normally elicits bilateral eye closure. Loss of this reflex with intact facial movement indicates ophthalmic division damage. Lesions of the motor component of V3 cause weakness of mastication muscles, resulting in jaw deviation toward the affected side when opening mouth (due to unopposed contralateral lateral pterygoid). With chronic denervation, atrophy of masseter and temporalis becomes visible. Herpes zoster can reactivate in the trigeminal ganglion, causing painful vesicular eruption in a dermatomal distribution. V1 involvement (herpes zoster ophthalmicus) requires ophthalmologic evaluation due to risk of keratitis and vision loss. Hutchinson's sign (vesicles on tip of nose from nasociliary nerve involvement) predicts higher risk of ocular complications. Central lesions affecting the spinal trigeminal tract and nucleus (as in Wallenberg syndrome) cause ipsilateral facial pain and temperature loss with characteristic "onion skin" distribution, sparing perioral region if only pars caudalis is affected.

Summary

The 12 pairs of cranial nerves represent a remarkably complex and clinically significant component of the human nervous system. Through their diverse sensory, motor, and autonomic functions, these nerves mediate essential processes including vision, olfaction, taste, hearing, balance, facial expression, eye movements, speech, swallowing, and visceral regulation. The anatomical organization of cranial nerves reflects their evolutionary heritage, developmental origins from distinct brainstem segments and branchial arches, and functional specialization for the unique requirements of the head and neck region.

Mastery of cranial nerve anatomy requires integration of multiple levels of understanding: the nuclear organization within the brainstem, the course of nerve fibers through the skull base, the peripheral distribution of branches, the functional components carried by each nerve, and the clinical manifestations of dysfunction. This knowledge forms the foundation for competent neurological examination and diagnosis, enabling clinicians to localize lesions with precision and to distinguish between peripheral neuropathies, brainstem nuclear lesions, and supranuclear pathology.

The Cerebellum

4

The cerebellum is a critical structure in the central nervous system responsible for motor coordination, balance, motor learning, and increasingly recognized cognitive functions. This chapter provides a comprehensive overview of cerebellar anatomy, physiology, and clinical correlations essential for understanding both normal function and pathological conditions.

Anatomical Organization

Gross Anatomical Divisions

The cerebellum is divided into three main lobes, each with distinct phylogenetic origins and functional specializations:

- *Anterior lobe* (paleocerebellum): Phylogenetically older, primarily involved in spinocerebellar functions
- *Posterior lobe* (neocerebellum): Phylogenetically newest, comprises the lateral hemispheres involved in motor planning and cognition
- *Flocculonodular lobe* (archicerebellum): Phylogenetically oldest, involved in vestibular function and balance

V. Yanamadala, *Essential Neuroanatomy*,
https://doi.org/10.1007/978-3-032-26877-8_4

Major Fissures

The cerebellar surface is characterized by several prominent fissures that divide the structure into distinct lobules:

- Primary fissure
- Posterior superior fissure
- Horizontal fissure
- Prepyramidal fissure
- Posterolateral fissure

Deep Cerebellar Nuclei

The cerebellum contains four pairs of deep nuclei that serve as the primary output structures, arranged from medial to lateral:

- *Fastigial nucleus* (most medial)
- *Globose nucleus*
- *Emboliform nucleus*
- *Dentate nucleus* (most lateral and largest)

Note: The globose and emboliform nuclei are collectively referred to as the interposed nuclei.

Medullary Substance (Corpus Medullare)

The medullary substance consists of white matter tracts deep to the cerebellar cortex. These tracts are continuous with the three cerebellar peduncles (superior, middle, and inferior) and contain fibers that interconnect cortical regions, carry Purkinje cell output to the deep nuclei, and convey recurrent fibers from the deep nuclei back to the cortex.

Cerebellar Cortex

The cerebellar cortex exhibits a uniform cytoarchitecture throughout, consisting of three distinct layers that are organized in a highly stereotyped manner. This consistent organization allows for efficient parallel processing of motor information (Fig. 4.1).

Cortical Layers

Molecular Layer

The outermost layer contains:

- *Stellate cells* (superficial): GABAergic interneurons that synapse onto Purkinje cell dendritic trees

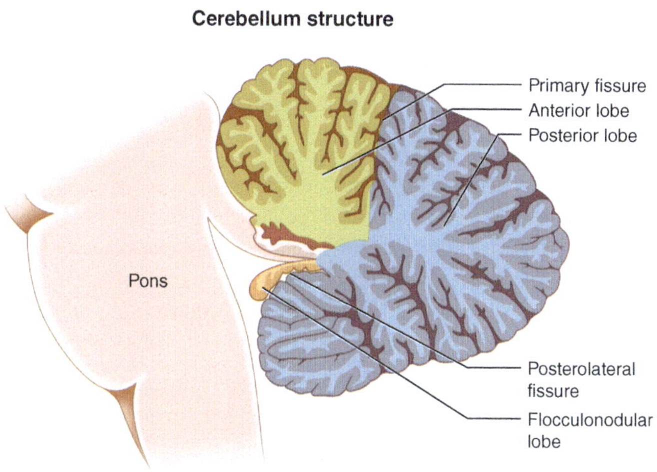

Fig. 4.1 Schematic lateral view of the cerebellum illustrating its lobar organization. The anterior lobe (green) is separated from the larger posterior lobe (blue) by the primary fissure, while the flocculonodular lobe is demarcated inferiorly by the posterolateral fissure. The relationship of the cerebellar peduncles to the pons is shown anteriorly

- *Basket cells* (deep): GABAergic interneurons that synapse onto Purkinje cell bodies, forming characteristic basket-like arrangements
- *Dendritic and axonal arborizations* from Purkinje cells and granule cells

Purkinje Cell Layer

This single-cell-thick layer contains the cell bodies of Purkinje cells, which are the sole output neurons of the cerebellar cortex. Each Purkinje cell possesses an extensive, planar dendritic tree that extends into the molecular layer.

Granular Layer

The innermost layer contains densely packed granule cell bodies, Golgi cell bodies, and specialized synaptic structures called glomeruli. This layer receives the majority of afferent input to the cerebellar cortex.

Cortical Cell Types

Purkinje Cells

Purkinje cells are the principal neurons of the cerebellar cortex and provide the sole output from the cortex to the deep cerebellar nuclei. A subset of Purkinje cells also sends output directly to the vestibular nuclei. These large neurons are characterized by their extensive, fan-shaped dendritic trees that lie in a single plane perpendicular to the long axis of the cerebellar folia. Purkinje cells are surrounded by specialized astrocyte satellite cells called Golgi epithelial cells, also known as Bergmann cells.

Granule Cells

Granule cells are the most numerous neurons in the human brain, with key characteristics:

- Approximately 5 μm in diameter, making them among the smallest neurons in the nervous system
- Number approximately 10^{10} in the human brain (out of a total of 10^{11} neurons)

- *The only glutamatergic (excitatory) cells in the cerebellar cortex*
- Receive all mossy fiber input to the cortex and relay this information via their axons (parallel fibers) to other cortical neurons

Basket Cells

Basket cells are GABAergic inhibitory interneurons that form distinctive basket-like structures around Purkinje cell somata. Their axons wrap around the Purkinje cell body and proximal dendrites, providing powerful inhibitory control.

Bergmann Cells (Golgi Epithelial Cells)

Bergmann cells are specialized radial glial cells that serve as satellite cells for Purkinje neurons. Their processes extend from the Purkinje cell layer through the molecular layer to the pial surface.

Bergmann gliosis: When Purkinje cells die, Bergmann cells proliferate to fill the space. Notably, the basket cell axonal fibers remain intact, creating the pathognomonic finding of "empty baskets" on histological examination—a diagnostic marker of Purkinje cell loss.

Stellate Cells

Stellate cells are GABAergic inhibitory interneurons located in the superficial molecular layer. They form inhibitory synapses onto the dendritic trees of Purkinje cells, providing dendritic inhibition.

Golgi Cells

Golgi cells are GABAergic inhibitory interneurons located in the granular layer. They form inhibitory synapses onto granule cells within the glomeruli, participating in feedback inhibition circuits that modulate granule cell activity.

Afferent Fibers

The cerebellar cortex receives two main types of afferent fibers—climbing fibers and mossy fibers—along with several modulatory inputs from monoaminergic and cholinergic systems. These afferent systems provide the cerebellum with information from diverse sources throughout the nervous system.

Climbing Fibers

Climbing fibers are glutamatergic excitatory fibers that originate from the contralateral inferior olivary nucleus and accessory olivary nuclei. Key features include:

- Each climbing fiber synapses directly onto a single Purkinje cell in the adult, arborizing extensively along the dendritic tree in a vine-like manner (hence the name "climbing" fiber).
- Early in the development, climbing fibers synapse onto multiple Purkinje cells; however, in adult humans, there is a one-to-one correspondence between climbing fibers and Purkinje cells.
- Climbing fibers synapse exclusively onto the smooth dendritic shaft, not onto dendritic spines.
- These fibers primarily target the paravermal zone and lateral hemispheres.
- Minor collaterals pass from each climbing fiber to nearby Purkinje cells.
- Some climbing fiber collaterals also synapse with granule cells and Golgi cells in the granular layer.

Mossy Fibers

Mossy fibers arise from multiple sources and provide the majority of afferent input to the cerebellum:

- *Sources:* Vestibular nuclei, spinocerebellar tracts, pontine nuclei, and recurrent fibers from the deep cerebellar nuclei
- *Targets:* Synapse onto granule cells and Golgi cells
- *Structure:* Mossy fibers give off terminal rosettes in the granular layer, which form specialized synaptic complexes called glomeruli

Glomerular structure: Each glomerulus consists of a mossy fiber rosette surrounded by approximately 20 interdigitating dendrites from granule and Golgi cells. The entire structure is encapsulated by a glial lamella formed by lamellar astrocytes, creating an isolated microenvironment for synaptic transmission.

Parallel Fibers

Parallel fibers are the axons of granule cells and represent the intrinsic processing pathway of the cerebellar cortex:

- Axons ascend vertically from the granular layer into the molecular layer, where they bifurcate.
- The bifurcated axons run horizontally through the molecular layer, parallel to one another and parallel to the long axis of the cerebellar folia.
- Parallel fibers synapse with all cerebellar cortical cell types, particularly forming en passant synapses onto dendritic spines of Purkinje cells.
- *Critical spatial organization:* Parallel fibers are orthogonal to (perpendicular to) the plane of Purkinje cell dendritic trees, allowing each parallel fiber to contact multiple Purkinje cells in sequence.

Modulatory Afferent Systems

Noradrenergic Fibers

Fibers from the locus coeruleus provide noradrenergic innervation to all cerebellar cell types. At low threshold levels, noradrenergic signaling through β1 receptors enhances GABA-mediated inhibition and independently hyperpolarizes target cells, modulating overall cerebellar excitability.

Dopaminergic Fibers

Fibers from the substantia nigra pars compacta (SN_C) and ventral tegmental area (VTA) provide dopaminergic innervation to the cerebellum. The precise functional role of these projections remains under investigation.

Serotonergic Fibers

Fibers from the raphe nuclei provide serotonergic innervation to all cells of the cerebellum except Purkinje cells, contributing to the modulation of cerebellar processing.

Cholinergic Fibers

Fibers from the pedunculopontine nucleus, and possibly some vestibular fibers, provide cholinergic innervation to cerebellar structures, though the complete functional significance remains to be fully elucidated.

Functional Divisions of the Cerebellum

The cerebellum can be functionally divided into three major regions based on their connectivity patterns, phylogenetic development, and clinical manifestations. Each division receives distinct inputs, projects to specific deep nuclei, and subserves different aspects of motor and vestibular control.

Vestibulocerebellum

Anatomical components: Flocculonodular lobe and uvula.

Vascular supply: Posterior inferior cerebellar artery (PICA).

Primary functions: Equilibrium, balance, and regulation of slow eye movements (including modulation of the vestibuloocular reflex and its cancellation).

Input Pathways

- Primary vestibular afferents from Scarpa's ganglia
- Secondary vestibular fibers from vestibular nuclei
- Olivocerebellar tracts from the inferior olivary complex

Note: Some secondary vestibular fibers also pass directly to the fastigial nucleus, bypassing the cortex.

Output Pathways

The cerebellar cortex of the vestibulocerebellum sends output to the fastigial and interposed nuclei. Additionally, some Purkinje cells project directly to the vestibular nuclei, making this the only region of the cerebellum with direct extracerebellar output from the cortex.

Clinical Correlation: Archicerebellar Syndrome

Medulloblastomas frequently arise in the roof of the caudal fourth ventricle in children, causing damage to the flocculonodular lobe. This results in loss of equilibrium with characteristic features: broad-based staggering gait, tendency to sway and fall (often with Romberg's sign positive), and truncal ataxia. Patients typically exhibit difficulty maintaining balance while standing or walking, even though limb coordination may be relatively preserved.

Spinocerebellum (Spinobulbocerebellum)

Anatomical components: Vermal and paravermal regions.

Vascular supply: Superior cerebellar artery (SCA).

Primary functions:

- *Paravermal regions:* Generate correcting signals for adjusting limb movements based on current position and desired targets
- *Vermal regions:* Control postural adjustment and axial musculature

Input Pathways

- Spinocerebellar tracts (dorsal and ventral)
- Cuneocerebellar tracts
- Rostral spinocerebellar tracts
- Trigeminocerebellar tracts (primarily from spinal nucleus of V—pars oralis and pars interpolaris)
- Fibers from the pontine and medullary reticular formation

- Pontocerebellar tracts
- Olivocerebellar tracts

Additionally, the spinocerebellum receives visual information from the visual cortex and superior colliculus via dorsolateral pontine nuclei, and auditory information from auditory cortex and inferior colliculus via other pontine nuclei.

Somatotopic Organization

The spinocerebellum contains three fractured somatotopic maps:

- One ipsilateral map in the anterior lobe
- Two bilateral maps in the posterior lobe

Within these maps: the head representation is closest to the primary fissure, the trunk is closest to the midline, and the legs are positioned most anteriorly.

Output Pathways

The cerebellar cortex of the spinocerebellum sends output to the fastigial nucleus (from vermal regions) and interposed nuclei (globose and emboliform; from paravermal regions).

Clinical Correlation: Anterior Lobe Syndrome

Chronic alcoholism with associated malnutrition causes characteristic degeneration of the vermis and paravermal zones, typically starting in the anterior lobes and progressing posteriorly (Fig. 4.2). Since the leg representations are located most anteriorly, the initial symptoms predominantly affect the lower extremities: broad-based staggering gait and lower limb ataxia. This may manifest on imaging as superior vermal atrophy. Upper extremity function is often relatively preserved in early stages.

Cerebrocerebellum (Neocerebellum)

Anatomical components: Lateral hemispheres.

Vascular supply: Superior cerebellar artery (SCA) and anterior inferior cerebellar artery (AICA).

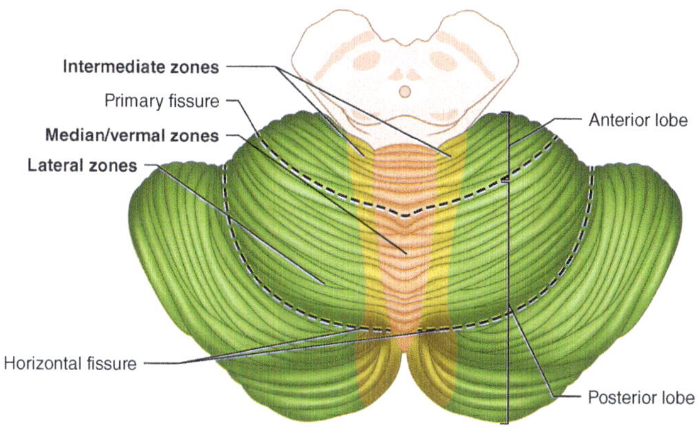

Fig. 4.2 Anterior view of the cerebellum demonstrating the transverse (lobular) and longitudinal (zonal) organization. The vermis and paravermian regions constitute the median/vermal and intermediate zones respectively, while the lateral hemispheres form the lateral zones. The primary fissure separates the anterior and posterior lobes superiorly, and the horizontal fissure divides the posterior lobe. The pons and superior cerebellar peduncles are visible superiorly

Primary functions: Planning and programming of voluntary movements, particularly learned, skillful movements that become more rapid, precise, and automatic with practice. Increasingly recognized for involvement in cognitive functions including attention, language, and working memory through connections with association cortex.

Input Pathways

- Cortical input via pontine nuclei (corticopontocerebellar pathway)

The corticopontocerebellar pathway represents a massive information channel:

- The majority of cerebral peduncle fibers terminate in the pontine nuclei
- Pontine nuclei contain approximately 12 million neurons on each side

- Pontine nuclei project to virtually all parts of the contralateral cerebellar cortex, with the exception of the flocculonodular lobe
- Input predominates from motor cortex, premotor cortex, somatosensory cortex, and association areas of the cerebral cortex
- Olivocerebellar tracts from the inferior olivary complex

Output Pathways

The cerebellar cortex of the cerebrocerebellum sends output exclusively to the dentate nuclei, which project to the motor and premotor cortex via the ventrolateral thalamus.

Clinical Correlation: Neocerebellar Syndrome

Damage to the lateral hemispheres produces a constellation of motor deficits, all occurring ipsilateral to the lesion:

- *Hypotonia*: Decreased muscle tone
- *Asynergia*: Inappropriate coordination of the direction, amplitude, and range of muscle contraction during complex movements
- *Hyporeflexia*: Decreased deep tendon reflexes
- *Pendular reflexes*: Excessive swinging of limbs following reflex testing due to hypotonia
- *Dysmetria*: Inability to judge distance or range of movement, resulting in overshooting or undershooting targets
- *Intention tremor*: Tremor that appears during voluntary movement, particularly as the target is approached (in contrast to Parkinsonian resting tremor)
- *Dysdiadochokinesia*: Inability to perform rapid alternating movements
- *Decomposition of movements*: Inability to coordinate complex movements requiring multiple sequential components; movements become broken into individual steps
- *Rebound phenomenon*: Inability to check movement quickly; if resistance is suddenly released, the limb may strike the patient or nearby objects

- *Scanning speech*: Ataxic dysarthria with irregular cadence and separated syllables
- *Nystagmus*: Rhythmic involuntary eye movements

Deep Cerebellar Nuclei

The deep cerebellar nuclei serve as the primary output stations of the cerebellum, receiving inhibitory input from Purkinje cells of the overlying cortex and excitatory input from extracerebellar sources. The balance between these inputs determines the final output of the cerebellar system.

General Principles of Nuclear Organization

Inhibitory Purkinje cell input: All deep nuclei receive GABAergic inhibitory input from Purkinje cells of the overlying cerebellar cortex
Excitatory extracerebellar input: All nuclei receive direct excitatory input from extracerebellar sources, providing tonic facilitation that opposes the GABAergic inhibitory input
Recurrent collaterals: All deep nuclei send recurrent efferent fibers back to the cerebellar cortex, where they synapse with granule cells, creating feedback loops

Important principle: Extracerebellar inputs to the deep nuclei are largely crossed, reflecting the general principle that the cerebellum is crossed with respect to the rest of the CNS but ipsilateral with respect to the body.

Dentate Nucleus

The largest and most lateral of the deep nuclei, the dentate nucleus receives input from the lateral hemispheres (cerebrocerebellum) and provides the major output pathway for motor planning and cognitive functions.

Extracerebellar inputs:

- Pontine nuclei
- Principal inferior olivary nucleus
- Trigeminal sensory nucleus
- Locus coeruleus
- Reticulotegmental nucleus (bilateral)
- Raphe nuclei

Interposed Nuclei (Globose and Emboliform)

The interposed nuclei, consisting of the globose (medial) and emboliform (lateral) nuclei, receive input from the paravermal regions of the spinocerebellum and participate in limb movement control.

Extracerebellar inputs:

- Medial accessory olivary nucleus
- Dorsal accessory olivary nucleus

Additionally, the emboliform nucleus receives fibers from the red nucleus, which are reciprocal to its output projections to the red nucleus, forming an important feedback loop.

Fastigial Nucleus

The most medial of the deep nuclei, the fastigial nucleus receives input from the vermal regions and flocculonodular lobe. It plays a crucial role in balance, posture, and axial motor control.

Extracerebellar inputs:

- Medial accessory olive (dorsomedial cell column and nucleus β)
- Bilateral input from medial and inferior vestibular nuclei (group x cells)

- Nucleus prepositus hypoglossi
- Dorsal paramedian reticular nuclei
- Locus coeruleus

Efferent Pathways from Deep Cerebellar Nuclei

The deep cerebellar nuclei project to various targets in the brainstem, thalamus, and spinal cord. These efferent pathways course through the three cerebellar peduncles and ultimately influence motor systems throughout the neuraxis.

Dentate Nucleus Efferents

The dentate nucleus projects primarily through the superior cerebellar peduncle:

- Fibers exit via the superior cerebellar peduncle
- Decussate completely in the caudal midbrain at the level of the inferior colliculus
- Project to the contralateral parvocellular red nucleus (dentatorubral tract)
- Continue to the contralateral ventrolateral (VL) nucleus of the thalamus, which projects to motor and premotor cortex (dentatothalamocortical pathway)

Interposed Nuclei Efferents

The interposed nuclei (globose and emboliform) also project through the superior cerebellar peduncle:

- Fibers exit via the superior cerebellar peduncle
- Decussate in the caudal midbrain
- Project to the contralateral magnocellular red nucleus, which gives rise to the rubrospinal tract
- Also project to the contralateral VL thalamus

Fastigial Nucleus Efferents

The fastigial nucleus has a unique bilateral projection pattern via the juxtarestiform body (medial portion of the inferior cerebellar peduncle):

Ipsilateral projections:

- Exit through the ipsilateral juxtarestiform body to ipsilateral vestibular nuclei and reticular formation

Contralateral projections:

- Cross the midline within the cerebellum
- Loop over the contralateral superior cerebellar peduncle as the uncinate fasciculus (hook bundle)
- Descend in the contralateral juxtarestiform body to vestibular nuclei and reticular formation

This bilateral pattern allows the fastigial nucleus to influence bilateral axial and proximal musculature for posture and balance.

Mollaret's Triangle (Guillain-Mollaret Triangle)

Mollaret's triangle is an important anatomical circuit connecting the cerebellum, red nucleus, and inferior olivary complex. Lesions in this circuit can produce palatal myoclonus and hypertrophic degeneration of the inferior olive.

The three components of the triangle:

- *First limb:* Dentate nucleus to contralateral parvocellular red nucleus via the dentatorubral tract (through superior cerebellar peduncle)
- *Second limb:* Parvocellular red nucleus to ipsilateral inferior olivary complex via the central tegmental tract (containing rubroolivary fibers)

- *Third limb:* Inferior olivary complex to contralateral cerebellar cortex via climbing fibers, which then influence the dentate nucleus through Purkinje cell axons

Functions of the Cerebellum

The cerebellum contributes to a wide range of motor and non-motor functions. While traditionally viewed primarily as a motor structure, accumulating evidence demonstrates important roles in cognitive and emotional processing as well.

Motor Coordination

The cerebellum coordinates voluntary muscle movements, ensuring smooth, precise, and accurate motor actions. It fine-tunes motor commands from the motor cortex by continuously comparing intended movements with actual performance, adjusts motor output to compensate for errors in real-time, and helps maintain appropriate muscle tone. This function is critical for all skilled voluntary movements.

Balance and Posture

The flocculonodular lobe and the vermis are crucial for equilibrium and postural control. The cerebellum integrates vestibular input (information about head position and movement) with proprioceptive feedback from the body to make continuous adjustments to posture and gait. This allows for maintenance of balance during static positions and dynamic movements.

Motor Learning

The cerebellum plays a central role in motor learning, particularly in the acquisition and refinement of skilled movements such as learning to ride a bicycle, play a musical instrument, or perform athletic skills. Through practice, the cerebellum helps automate complex motor sequences, allowing them to be performed with increasing speed and accuracy while requiring less conscious attention.

Cerebellar Learning Mechanisms

The cerebellum can send signals to the frontal motor cortex to affect general movement patterns and to the prefrontal cortex to affect the processing of signs and symbols, suggesting a role in cognitive learning. Additionally, the cerebellum modulates the vestibuloocular reflex and optokinetic reflex, allowing adaptive changes in eye movements. These learning processes are possibly encoded within the interactions between climbing fibers, Purkinje cells, and mossy fibers, as these synaptic connections demonstrate plasticity over time. Electrophysiology studies have demonstrated that appropriate stimulation patterns result in long-term potentiation and depression at these synapses, providing a cellular mechanism for cerebellar learning.

Cognitive and Emotional Processing

Although traditionally associated primarily with motor control, accumulating evidence demonstrates that the cerebellum also contributes to cognitive functions including attention, language processing, working memory, and executive function. The cerebellum has extensive anatomical connections to regions of the prefrontal cortex via thalamocortical pathways. Furthermore, the cerebellum is involved in emotional regulation through its connections to limbic structures, contributing to the modulation of emotional responses and affective states.

Clinical Relevance: Disorders of the Cerebellum

Damage to the cerebellum results in a variety of neurological deficits that reflect the specific regions and functions affected. Understanding cerebellar clinical syndromes is essential for anatomical localization and diagnosis.

Cerebellar Signs and Symptoms

Ataxia

Ataxia is a disorder characterized by a lack of coordination and unsteady movements, commonly seen in patients with cerebellar lesions. Cerebellar ataxia can affect the limbs (appendicular ataxia), trunk (truncal ataxia), and speech (ataxic dysarthria). Cerebellar ataxia is most commonly associated with damage to the posterior lobe and vermis.

Dysmetria

Dysmetria represents an inability to judge accurately the distance or range of a movement, resulting in overshooting (hypermetria) or undershooting (hypometria) of intended targets. This deficit is particularly evident during finger-to-nose and heel-to-shin testing. Dysmetria occurs when the spinocerebellum (particularly the paravermal regions) is impaired.

Intention Tremor

Intention tremor is a tremor that occurs during voluntary movements, becoming more pronounced as the individual approaches a target. This contrasts sharply with Parkinsonian resting tremor, which is most prominent at rest and diminishes with voluntary movement. Intention tremor is a hallmark sign of damage to the cerebellar hemispheres or dentate nucleus.

Nystagmus

Nystagmus consists of involuntary, rapid, rhythmic eye movements that may occur with vestibulocerebellar lesions affecting the flocculonodular lobe. The nystagmus may be horizontal, vertical, or rotatory depending on the specific structures involved.

Neoplastic Conditions

Medulloblastoma

Medulloblastoma is a malignant cerebellar tumor that typically arises in the vermis and occurs predominantly during childhood. These tumors characteristically originate in the roof of the fourth ventricle and can rapidly expand to fill the ventricular space, causing obstruction of CSF flow and resulting in non-communicating hydrocephalus. Clinical presentation includes symptoms of increased intracranial pressure (headache, nausea, vomiting) along with truncal ataxia and balance difficulties due to vermal involvement.

Cerebellar Pilocytic Astrocytoma

Pilocytic astrocytoma is a typically benign, slow-growing tumor most commonly seen in young children. These tumors often arise in the cerebellar hemispheres and are characterized by cystic components with an enhancing mural nodule on imaging. Surgical resection is usually curative, with excellent long-term prognosis when complete removal is achieved.

Congenital Malformations: Chiari Malformations

Chiari malformations represent a spectrum of congenital anomalies characterized by structural defects at the craniocervical junction. These malformations involve abnormal positioning of the cerebellum and, in some cases, the brainstem relative to the foramen magnum.

Chiari Type I Malformation

Type I involves the extension of the cerebellar tonsils (the inferior portion of the cerebellar hemispheres) through the foramen magnum, without involving the brainstem. Normally, only the spinal cord passes through this opening. Type I is the most common form of Chiari malformation and represents the only type that can be acquired (though most cases are congenital). Clinical features:

- Many patients remain asymptomatic
- Often first discovered incidentally during imaging for other conditions
- Typically presents in adolescence or adulthood
- When symptomatic, may cause headaches (particularly with Valsalva), neck pain, balance problems, and rarely syringomyelia

Chiari Type II Malformation (Arnold-Chiari Malformation)

Type II, also called classic Chiari malformation, involves the extension of both cerebellar tissue and brainstem structures through the foramen magnum. This is a more severe malformation with several characteristic features:

- Herniation of cerebellar vermis and brainstem through foramen magnum
- The cerebellar vermis may be incomplete or absent
- Almost invariably accompanied by myelomeningocele (a form of spina bifida)
- Commonly associated with hydrocephalus

Myelomeningocele occurs when the spinal canal and backbone fail to close completely before birth, causing the spinal cord and its protective membranes to protrude through a sac-like opening in the back. This typically results in partial or complete paralysis of the body below the level of the spinal opening. The term Arnold-Chiari malformation (named after the pioneering researchers Julius Arnold and Hans Chiari) specifically refers to Type II malformations.

Chiari Type III Malformation

Type III is the most serious form of Chiari malformation, characterized by severe herniation of posterior fossa contents:

- The cerebellum and brainstem protrude or herniate through the foramen magnum into the cervical spinal canal
- Part of the fourth ventricle may also protrude through the foramen magnum
- In rare instances, the herniated tissue can cause an occipital encephalocele—a pouch-like structure protruding from the back of the head or neck that contains brain tissue and meninges
- The covering of the brain or spinal cord (meninges) can also protrude through abnormal openings in the skull or spine
- Results in severe neurological deficits and is often incompatible with life

Chiari Type IV Malformation

Type IV involves an incomplete or underdeveloped cerebellum, a condition known as cerebellar hypoplasia. This is an extremely rare form with distinctive characteristics: the cerebellar tonsils are located further down into the spinal canal than normal, significant portions of the cerebellum are absent or severely underdeveloped, and portions of the skull and spinal cord may be visible through developmental defects. The severe cerebellar hypoplasia results in profound neurological impairment.

Chiari Type 0 Malformation (Controversial)

Some researchers have proposed a Type 0 classification, though this remains under debate in the medical community. In this putative form, patients exhibit clinical symptoms characteristic of Chiari malformation (such as headaches, particularly with Valsalva maneuver) without radiographic evidence of cerebellar tonsillar herniation through the foramen magnum. The existence and clinical significance of this category continue to be subjects of ongoing investigation.

Summary

The cerebellum represents a highly organized structure with consistent cytoarchitecture throughout its cortex, enabling sophisticated parallel processing of motor and cognitive information. Understanding its anatomical organization, functional divisions, connectivity patterns, and clinical manifestations is essential for neurological diagnosis and localization of pathology. This foundation provides the basis for understanding both normal cerebellar function in motor coordination, learning, and cognition and the diverse clinical presentations resulting from cerebellar dysfunction.

The Diencephalon

5

Introduction

The diencephalon is a major division of the forebrain that plays a pivotal role in relaying sensory and motor signals to the cerebral cortex, regulating autonomic functions, and maintaining homeostasis. Situated deep within the brain, immediately rostral to the brainstem and encased by the cerebral hemispheres, the diencephalon contains structures critical for sensory processing, motor control, emotional regulation, and endocrine function.

The diencephalon is anatomically positioned between the midbrain inferiorly and the cerebral cortex superiorly. This strategic location enables it to serve as an integrative hub for ascending sensory pathways and descending motor commands. The structures within the diencephalon work in concert to process information, coordinate responses, and maintain physiological equilibrium.

Major Divisions of the Diencephalon

The diencephalon comprises four principal structural and functional divisions (Fig. 5.1):

V. Yanamadala, *Essential Neuroanatomy*,
https://doi.org/10.1007/978-3-032-26877-8_5

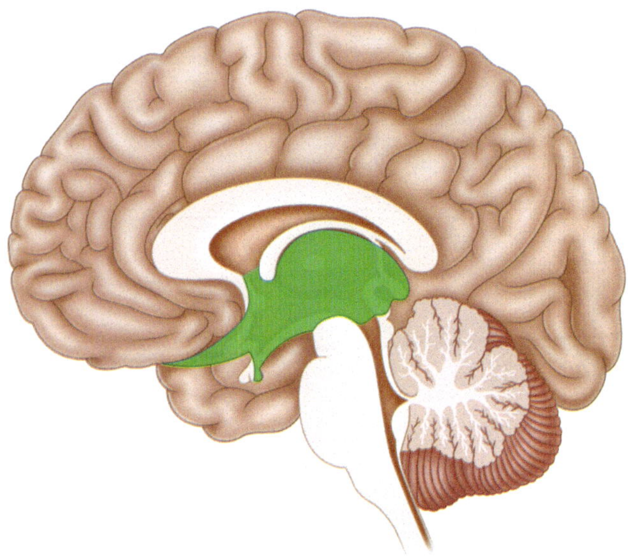

Fig. 5.1 Sagittal section of the brain with the diencephalon highlighted in green, illustrating its central position between the cerebral hemispheres and the brainstem. The diencephalon encompasses the thalamus, hypothalamus, subthalamus, and epithalamus and is bounded superiorly by the corpus callosum, anteriorly by the interventricular foramen, and inferiorly by the junction with the midbrain tegmentum

- Thalamus: The primary sensory relay nucleus
- Hypothalamus: The master regulator of autonomic and endocrine function
- Epithalamus: Including the pineal gland and habenular nuclei
- Subthalamus: Including the subthalamic nucleus and associated motor structures

Each division possesses distinct anatomical characteristics and functional specializations, yet they demonstrate significant interconnectivity and functional overlap in regulating complex neural processes.

The Thalamus

Overview and General Organization

The thalamus is a large, bilaterally paired structure occupying the central region of the diencephalon. Functionally characterized as the brain's "relay station," the thalamus contains numerous distinct nuclei that process and transmit information between subcortical structures and the cerebral cortex. With the notable exception of olfactory information, virtually all sensory modalities pass through thalamic nuclei en route to cortical processing centers (Fig. 5.2).

Structural Organization

The internal medullary lamina, a Y-shaped sheet of myelinated fibers, divides the thalamus into distinct nuclear groups. The external medullary lamina covers the lateral thalamic surface and separates the lateral nuclear group from the thalamic reticular nucleus. This architectural organization facilitates the functional specialization observed among thalamic nuclei.

Thalamic neurons exist in two distinct functional states that significantly influence information transmission:

- *Tonic mode*: The normal operational state during wakefulness, characterized by faithful transmission of input signals
- *Burst mode*: A hyperpolarized state where small depolarizations activate slow voltage-gated calcium channels, producing prolonged depolarizations. During sleep, increased numbers of thalamic neurons enter burst mode, reducing signal transmission capacity

Thalamic output is modulated by three primary sources: the cortical areas to which nuclei project, the thalamic reticular nucleus, and diffuse ascending cholinergic, noradrenergic, and serotonergic pathways from the brainstem.

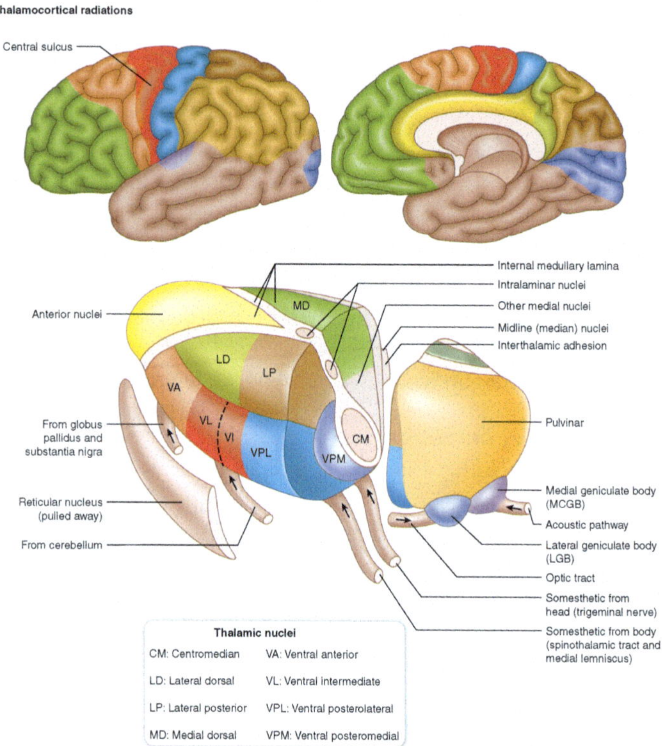

Fig. 5.2 The thalamic nuclei and their thalamocortical radiations (Netter). Upper panels show color-coded projections of individual thalamic nuclei to their corresponding cortical territories on lateral and medial brain surfaces. The lower panel depicts a three-dimensional dissection of the thalamus illustrating the major nuclear groups—including the anterior nuclei, lateral dorsal (LD), lateral posterior (LP), ventral anterior (VA), ventral intermediate (VI), ventral lateral (VL), ventral posterolateral (VPL), ventral posteromedial (VPM), centromedian (CM), mediodorsal (MD), and pulvinar—along with their principal afferent inputs from the cerebellum, globus pallidus, substantia nigra, spinothalamic tract, medial lemniscus, trigeminal nerve, reticular nucleus, medial geniculate body (auditory pathway), and lateral geniculate body (optic tract)

Functional Classification of Thalamic Nuclei

Thalamic nuclei are functionally categorized as either relay nuclei or association nuclei. Relay nuclei project predominantly to cortical layers III, IV, V, and VI, while association nuclei project mainly to cortical layer I. This differential projection pattern reflects distinct roles in cortical processing.

Specific Thalamic Nuclei and Their Connections

Anterior Nuclear Group

The anterior group includes the anteroventral, anterodorsal, and anteriomedial nuclei, which serve as relay nuclei for the limbic system. These nuclei play crucial roles in emotion processing and recent memory formation.

Afferent Connections:

- Mamillary bodies via the mammillothalamic tract
- Temporal cortex and hippocampus (primarily presubicular fibers) via the fornix
- Raphe nuclei, pedunculopontine nucleus, and laterodorsal tegmental nuclei

Efferent connections: Project to the cingulate gyrus (Brodmann areas 23, 24, 32) via the anterior limb of the internal capsule.

Dorsomedial Nucleus

The dorsomedial nucleus functions as an association nucleus involved in affect, foresight, and emotional processing. It consists of three subdivisions:

Pars Magnocellularis:

- Receives input from the amygdala, hypothalamus (via hypothalamothalamic fibers), basal forebrain (substantia innominata and basal nucleus of Meynert), temporal cortex, and frontal orbital gyri
- Projects to the basal nucleus of Meynert and prefrontal cortex

Pars Parvocellularis

- Receives fibers from the entire prefrontal cortex
- Projects reciprocally to the prefrontal cortex

Pars Multiformis (Paralaminaris)

- Receives fibers from the substantia nigra pars reticularis
- Efferent projections remain incompletely characterized

Midline Nuclei

The midline nuclei represent a rostral continuation of the midbrain periaqueductal gray matter, extending to form the interthalamic adhesion (massa intermedia).

Pulvinar

The pulvinar, comprising pars oralis, pars lateralis, pars medialis, and pars inferior, serves as the association nucleus for the parietal-occipital-temporal association cortex.

Afferent Connections:

- Parietal association cortex
- Ipsilateral superior colliculus (representing contralateral visual field), primarily to pars inferior
- Reciprocal connections with striate cortex

Efferent Connections:

- Parietal association cortex
- Retinotopic projections to visual association areas and striate cortex

Lateral Posterior Nucleus

The lateral posterior nucleus functions as an extension of the pulvinar with analogous connectivity and function in visual-spatial processing.

Lateral Dorsal Nucleus

This limbic association nucleus receives input from the hippocampus and projects to the cingulate gyrus and supralimbic regions of the parietal cortex.

Ventral Anterior Nucleus

The ventral anterior nucleus initiates and regulates motor activity. It consists of two subdivisions:

Pars Magnocellularis:

- Receives input from the substantia nigra pars reticularis
- Projects to premotor cortex (Brodmann area 6, anterior precentral gyrus)

Pars Parvocellularis:

- Receives input from the globus pallidus internus
- Projects to premotor cortex (Brodmann area 6)

Ventral Lateral Nucleus

The ventral lateral nucleus, including pars oralis, pars medialis, and pars caudalis, modulates motor activity.

- Receives input from deep cerebellar nuclei (and limited input from globus pallidus internus)
- Projects to the primary motor cortex (Brodmann area 4, posterior precentral gyrus) and premotor cortex (Brodmann area 6)

Ventral Posterolateral Nucleus

The ventral posterolateral nucleus, comprising pars oralis and pars caudalis, processes somatosensory information from the body.

- Receives input from the nucleus cuneatus, nucleus gracilis, and spinothalamic tracts
- Projects to postcentral gyrus (Brodmann areas 1–3) and primary motor cortex (VPL pars oralis)

Ventral Posteromedial Nucleus

This nucleus processes sensory information from the head and consists of two subdivisions:

Pars principalis: Processes touch, pressure, pain, thermal sensation, and proprioception from the head.

- Receives input from principal and spinal trigeminal nuclei
- Projects to inferolateral postcentral gyrus (Brodmann areas 1–3)

Pars parvocellularis: Processes gustatory information.

- Receives input from the ipsilateral nucleus solitarius and parabrachial nuclei
- Projects to the parietal operculum (Brodmann area 43)

Lateral Geniculate Nucleus

The lateral geniculate nucleus (LGN) serves as the primary relay for visual information. It consists of six layers: magnocellular layers 1 and 2 and parvocellular layers 3–6.

Retinal Input Organization:

- Layers 1, 4, and 6: Receive projections from contralateral retina
- Layers 2, 3, and 5: Receive projections from ipsilateral retina

Afferent Connections:

- Optic tract (approximately 10% of total LGN input)
- Visual cortex feedback (over 50% of total LGN input)

Efferent connections: Projects to primary visual cortex (Brodmann area 17) via geniculocalcarine radiations.

Cellular organization: The LGN contains three functional cell types:

- Parvocellular (X cells): Receive input from midget foveal ganglion cells
- Magnocellular (Y cells): Receive input from parasol peripheral ganglion cells
- Koniocellular (Z cells): Receive bistratified information and project to all cortical layers

Medial Geniculate Nucleus

The medial geniculate nucleus (MGN), comprising medial, dorsal, and ventral divisions, processes auditory information.

- Receives input from the inferior colliculus via the inferior brachium
- Projects to the primary auditory cortex (Brodmann area 41) via auditory (geniculotemporal) radiations

Posterior Intralaminar Group

The centromedian and parafascicular nuclei constitute the posterior intralaminar group. These nuclei play important roles in arousal, attention, and motor control.

Centromedian Nucleus:

- Receives input from the motor cortex and globus pallidus internus
- Projects to the putamen

Parafascicular Nucleus:

- Receives input from the globus pallidus internus
- Projects to the caudate nucleus

Anterior Intralaminar Group

The central medial, paracentral, and central lateral nuclei comprise the anterior intralaminar group. These nuclei receive input from the reticular formation and project diffusely to the cerebral cortex, contributing to arousal and consciousness.

Thalamic Reticular Nucleus

The thalamic reticular nucleus forms a thin shell around the lateral aspect of the thalamus. This GABAergic nucleus receives collaterals from thalamocortical and corticothalamic fibers and projects back to thalamic nuclei, providing inhibitory modulation of thalamic activity.

The Hypothalamus

Overview and Functional Significance

The hypothalamus, though comprising less than 1% of total brain mass, exerts profound influence over autonomic, endocrine, and behavioral functions. Positioned below the thalamus and forming the floor and inferior lateral walls of the third ventricle, the hypothalamus integrates neural and hormonal signals to maintain homeostasis.

Anatomical Organization

The hypothalamus is organized into distinct zones along both anterior-posterior and medial-lateral axes. This organization reflects functional specialization among hypothalamic nuclei.

Anterior-Posterior Organization

Preoptic Region (Anterior Hypothalamus):

Medial preoptic nucleus: Regulates sexual behavior and gonadotropin-releasing hormone (GnRH) secretion

Lateral preoptic nucleus: Produces GnRH

Median preoptic nucleus: Regulates osmotic homeostasis

Preoptic periventricular nucleus: Regulates temperature, involved in thermoregulation

Suprachiasmatic nucleus: Serves as the primary circadian pacemaker, receiving direct retinal input via the retinohypothalamic tract

Paraventricular nucleus: Contains magnocellular neurons producing oxytocin and antidiuretic hormone (ADH), and parvocellular neurons producing corticotropin-releasing hormone (CRH) and thyrotropin-releasing hormone (TRH)

Supraoptic nucleus: Produces oxytocin and ADH

Anterior hypothalamic nucleus: Regulates heat dissipation and parasympathetic tone

Supraoptic commissures: Include the anterior commissure, dorsal supraoptic commissure (Ganser's commissure), and ventral supraoptic commissure (Gudden's commissure)

Tuberal Region (Middle Hypothalamus):

Dorsomedial nucleus: Regulates blood pressure, heart rate, and gastrointestinal function

Ventromedial nucleus: Functions as a satiety center; lesions produce hyperphagia and obesity

Arcuate nucleus: Produces releasing and inhibiting hormones that regulate anterior pituitary function; contains neurons sensitive to leptin and ghrelin

Posterior Region (Mammillary Bodies and Posterior Hypothalamus):

Posterior hypothalamic nucleus: Regulates heat production, blood pressure, and sympathetic tone

Lateral hypothalamic area: Functions as a feeding center; lesions produce aphagia

Mammillary bodies: Comprise medial and lateral mammillary nuclei; receive input from hippocampus via fornix and project to anterior thalamic nuclei via mammillothalamic tract; critical for memory formation

Medial-Lateral Organization

Periventricular Zone:

Located adjacent to the third ventricle, this zone contains small neurons that regulate anterior pituitary function through hypothalamic-releasing hormones.

Medial Zone:

The medial zone contains the majority of hypothalamic nuclei and is innervated by the fornix, which carries hippocampal projections.

Lateral Zone:

The lateral zone, innervated bidirectionally by the amygdala via the stria terminalis, contains several important nuclei:

- *Lateral nucleus*: May regulate thirst
- *Lateral preoptic nucleus*: Produces GnRH
- *Lateral tuberal nuclei*: Function as a feeding center
- *Tuberomammillary nucleus*: Serves as the source of histaminergic fibers projecting widely to cerebral cortex and thalamus; plays a critical role in the sleep-wake cycle

Hypothalamic Connections

Major Afferent Pathways

- *Medial forebrain bundle*: Conveys fibers from septal nuclei, paraolfactory area, and striatum to hypothalamus
- *Thalamohypothalamic fibers*: Originate from medial and midline thalamic nuclei
- *Fornix*: Carries hippocampal projections to mammillary bodies
- *Stria terminalis*: Conveys amygdalar projections
- *Ventral amygdalofugal pathway*: Provides direct amygdalar input
- *Pallidohypothalamic fibers*: Project from globus pallidus internus to ventromedial hypothalamic nucleus
- *Inferior mammillary peduncle*: Carries fibers from midbrain tegmentum
- *Retinohypothalamic tract*: Less than 1% of retinal ganglion cells project directly to suprachiasmatic nucleus bilaterally; these specialized ganglion cells utilize melanopsin as their light detector
- *Left insular cortex*: Drives anterior nucleus parasympathetic pathways
- *Right insular cortex*: Drives posterior nucleus sympathetic pathways

Major Efferent Pathways

- *Medial forebrain bundle*: Distributes hypothalamic projections to forebrain structures
- *Fornix*: Carries projections from mammillary bodies to hippocampus
- *Hypothalamohypophyseal tract*: Conveys axons from supraoptic and paraventricular nuclei carrying Herring bodies (containing ADH and oxytocin) through the infundibulum to the posterior pituitary
- *Hypophyseotropic tract*: Projects from arcuate nucleus to median eminence, releasing anterior pituitary regulatory hormones into the hypothalamic-hypophyseal portal system
- *Hypothalamospinal tract*: Projects from hypothalamus to intermediolateral cell columns; descends in the lateral funiculus of the spinal cord
- *Hypothalamomedullary tract*: Provides autonomic control to brainstem parasympathetic nuclei

Functional Responses to Hypothalamic Stimulation

Experimental stimulation of hypothalamic regions produces distinct, reproducible physiological and behavioral responses:

Posterolateral Hypothalamus Activation:

- Activates stress response
- Increases sympathetic tone
- Increases aggression
- Increases hunger
- Increases body temperature

Anteromedial Hypothalamus Activation:

- Produces contentment
- Increases parasympathetic tone
- Increases passivity and satiety
- Decreases body temperature

Circumventricular Organs

Circumventricular organs are specialized regions with an attenuated blood-brain barrier, enabling direct sensing of circulating molecules. These structures include:

- *Vascular organ of the lamina terminalis*: Located in the midline hypothalamus
- *Median eminence*: Site of hypothalamic hormone release into portal circulation
- *Posterior pituitary*: Releases ADH and oxytocin into systemic circulation
- *Subfornical organ*: Monitors circulating angiotensin II
- *Area postrema*: Signals to nucleus ambiguus to regulate nausea and vomiting

The hypophyseal veins drain to the cavernous sinus, establishing venous return from the pituitary gland.

The Epithalamus

Overview and Components

The epithalamus is a small but functionally significant region located superior and posterior to the thalamus. It comprises the pineal gland and habenular nuclei, structures involved in circadian rhythm regulation and emotional processing.

Habenular Complex

The habenula is positioned rostrolateral to the pineal gland. The left and right habenular nuclei are connected by the habenular commissure.

Lateral Habenular Nucleus:

- Receives input from the globus pallidus internus, lateral hypothalamus, substantia innominata, lateral preoptic area, ventral tegmental area, and mesencephalic raphe nuclei
- Functions as an interface between limbic and motor systems
- Plays a role in reward processing and aversion

Medial Habenular Nucleus:

- Receives input from septal nuclei
- Functions as a limbic system relay
- Contains primarily cholinergic neurons

Habenular Connections

Stria medullaris: Carries afferent fibers from anterior thalamus, hypothalamus, septal nuclei, and forebrain to habenular nuclei. These fibers decussate in the habenular commissure. The stria medullaris courses medial to the medial division of the thalamus.

Habenulointerpeduncular tract (fasciculus retroflexus): Conveys efferent projections from habenular nuclei to the interpeduncular nucleus in the midbrain tegmentum. This tract passes through the parafascicular nucleus of the thalamus.

Pineal Gland

The pineal gland, also termed the epiphysis cerebri, functions as the primary source of melatonin, a hormone crucial for circadian rhythm regulation.

Hormonal Production

The pineal gland produces multiple bioactive substances:

- *Melatonin*: Synthesized during dark periods, regulates sleep-wake cycles
- *Serotonin*: Precursor for melatonin synthesis
- *Norepinephrine*: Released during sympathetic activation
- *Neuropeptides*: Including TRH, GnRH, and somatostatin

Light Input Pathway and Melatonin Regulation

The circadian regulation of melatonin synthesis involves a complex neural pathway:

- Retinal ganglion cells containing melanopsin project directly to the suprachiasmatic nucleus via the retinohypothalamic tract
- The suprachiasmatic nucleus processes light information and regulates circadian timing
- Hypothalamic projections modulate sympathetic nerves innervating the pineal gland
- Sympathetic stimulation increases melatonin synthesis
- Two key enzymes, N-acetyltransferase and hydroxyindole-O-methyltransferase, are upregulated during darkness, facilitating melatonin synthesis

Anatomical Landmark

Calcareous concretions (corpora arenacea or "brain sand") accumulate in the pineal gland with age, rendering it visible on radiological imaging and serving as a useful midline landmark for identifying mass effects and midline shift.

The Subthalamus

Overview and Function

The subthalamus occupies the region ventral to the thalamus and functions primarily as a component of the basal ganglia motor control circuitry. Key structures include the subthalamic nucleus, zona incerta, and rostral portions of the red nucleus and substantia nigra.

Subthalamic Nucleus

The subthalamic nucleus serves as a critical node in the basal ganglia circuit, essential for controlling voluntary movements. It modulates globus pallidus output and regulates motor activity through the indirect pathway.

Clinical Significance: Hemiballismus

Stroke affecting the subthalamic nucleus produces hemiballismus, a hyperkinetic movement disorder characterized by violent, flinging movements of the contralateral limbs. This disorder results from loss of the indirect pathway, leading to disinhibition of thalamic motor nuclei.

Associated Structures

Zona incerta: Represents a rostral continuation of the midbrain reticular formation. Located between the thalamus and subthalamic nucleus, the zona incerta lies directly inferior to the thalamic reticular nucleus.

Red nucleus (rostral portions): The rostral aspect of the red nucleus extends into the subthalamic region.

Substantia nigra (rostral portions): The rostral substantia nigra also extends into the subthalamic territory.

Vascular Supply of the Diencephalon

The diencephalon receives its arterial blood supply from multiple vessels, predominantly branches of the posterior cerebral artery and internal carotid artery systems. This dual supply provides some degree of collateral circulation but also creates vulnerability to specific vascular territories.

Major Arterial Supply

- *Thalamogeniculate arteries*: Arise from the posterior cerebral artery and supply the thalamus
- *Posterior communicating artery*: Provides collateral circulation between internal carotid and posterior cerebral artery systems, contributing to hypothalamic and thalamic blood supply
- *Posterior cerebral artery*: Supplies the epithalamus and portions of the thalamus

Clinical Correlation: Wernicke-Korsakoff Syndrome

Wernicke-Korsakoff syndrome results from thiamine (vitamin B1) deficiency, most commonly associated with chronic alcoholism. This condition produces selective infarction of specific diencephalic and brainstem structures:

- Mammillary bodies
- Dorsal median nucleus of the thalamus
- Oculomotor nucleus
- Dorsal motor nucleus of the vagus

The acute phase (Wernicke encephalopathy) presents with the classic triad of confusion, ataxia, and ophthalmoplegia. The chronic phase (Korsakoff syndrome) manifests as severe anterograde amnesia with confabulation. Prompt thiamine replacement can prevent progression to permanent memory impairment.

Summary

The diencephalon represents a critical integration center within the central nervous system, bridging subcortical and cortical structures while regulating essential physiological and behavioral functions. The thalamus serves as the primary relay for sensory and motor information, with highly organized nuclei projecting to specific cortical regions. The hypothalamus, despite its small size, exerts profound control over autonomic, endocrine, and homeostatic functions through its extensive connections with both neural and hormonal systems. The epithalamus regulates circadian rhythms and processes reward-related information through the pineal gland and habenular nuclei. The subthalamus plays an essential role in motor control as part of the basal ganglia circuitry.

Understanding diencephalic neuroanatomy is fundamental for medical professionals, as pathology affecting these structures produces diverse neurological, psychiatric, and endocrine manifestations. From movement disorders like hemiballismus and Parkinson's disease to memory impairments in Wernicke-Korsakoff syndrome, diencephalic dysfunction underlies numerous clinical conditions. Mastery of this anatomical region provides an essential foundation for clinical neuroscience and enables accurate diagnosis and management of neurological disorders.

The Basal Ganglia

6

Introduction

The basal ganglia constitute a collection of interconnected subcortical nuclei that are fundamental to the regulation of voluntary movement, motor learning, and various cognitive and emotional processes. These structures form complex circuits with the cerebral cortex and thalamus, creating feedback loops that fine-tune motor output and suppress unwanted movements. Dysfunction within the basal ganglia circuitry results in characteristic movement disorders that can be either hypokinetic (reduced movement) or hyperkinetic (excessive involuntary movements).

Major Components of the Basal Ganglia

The basal ganglia consist of several key structures, each contributing uniquely to motor and cognitive function (Fig. 6.1).

V. Yanamadala, *Essential Neuroanatomy*,
https://doi.org/10.1007/978-3-032-26877-8_6

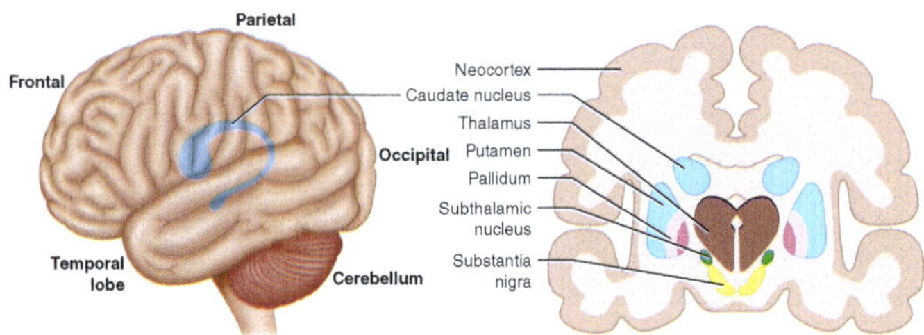

Fig. 6.1 Lateral view of the brain (left) and coronal section (right) illustrating the anatomical relationships of the basal ganglia. The coronal section identifies the caudate nucleus, putamen, pallidum (globus pallidus), thalamus, subthalamic nucleus, and substantia nigra within the context of the surrounding neocortex and white matter

Caudate Nucleus

The caudate nucleus is a large, C-shaped structure that, together with the putamen, forms the striatum. It is positioned along the lateral wall of the lateral ventricle and extends from the frontal horn posteriorly into the temporal lobe. The caudate nucleus receives extensive cortical input, particularly from the frontal lobe, and plays important roles in motor control, learning, memory, and cognitive processes such as planning movements and habit formation.

Putamen

The putamen represents the other major component of the striatum and is primarily involved in the control and regulation of movement, particularly the planning and execution of voluntary motor actions. The putamen works in close coordination with the caudate nucleus and maintains extensive connections with both the motor cortex and the thalamus. Together with the globus pallidus, the putamen forms the lenticular nucleus.

Globus Pallidus

The globus pallidus (also called the pallidum) is divided into two distinct segments with different functions:

External Segment (GPe)

The external segment modulates thalamic output and serves as an intermediate relay in the indirect pathway. It receives inhibitory GABAergic input from the striatum and provides inhibitory output to the subthalamic nucleus and internal segment of the globus pallidus.

Internal Segment (GPi)

The internal segment acts as one of the principal output structures of the basal ganglia, along with the substantia nigra pars reticulata. The GPi provides inhibitory GABAergic signals to the thalamus to regulate voluntary movement. The globus pallidus plays crucial roles in movement initiation, suppression of unwanted voluntary movements, and regulation of muscle tone.

Subthalamic Nucleus

The subthalamic nucleus (STN) is located ventral to the thalamus and is involved in modulating the activity of both the globus pallidus and the substantia nigra. Unlike most basal ganglia structures, the STN uses glutamate as its neurotransmitter and provides excitatory input to the GPi and substantia nigra pars reticulata. This excitatory influence can significantly affect motor output from the basal ganglia.

Substantia Nigra

The substantia nigra is a brainstem structure divided into two functionally distinct parts:

Pars Compacta (SNc)

The pars compacta contains dopaminergic neurons that provide crucial excitatory and modulatory input to the striatum, facilitating voluntary movement. The characteristic dark pigmentation of this region becomes apparent during adolescence and results from neuromelanin, which is formed from the dimerization of dopamine. This region is particularly important in the pathophysiology of Parkinson's disease, where progressive loss of dopamine-producing neurons leads to motor deficits including tremors, rigidity, and bradykinesia.

Pars Reticulata (SNr)

The pars reticulata functions similarly to the globus pallidus internus, sending inhibitory GABAergic signals to the thalamus and contributing to the regulation of motor activity.

Functional Anatomy and Neural Pathways

The basal ganglia operate through complex circuits involving feedback loops between the cortex, thalamus, and basal ganglia structures (Fig. 6.2). These circuits can be broadly categorized into direct and indirect pathways, which have opposing effects on motor output.

The Direct Pathway: Facilitation of Movement

The direct pathway facilitates voluntary movement by increasing thalamic output to the motor cortex. This pathway involves the following sequence:

- The cerebral cortex stimulates the striatum (caudate nucleus and putamen).
- The striatum inhibits the globus pallidus internus (GPi).
- Inhibition of the GPi decreases its inhibitory output to the thalamus.
- The thalamus becomes disinhibited and more active, stimulating the motor cortex to initiate movement.

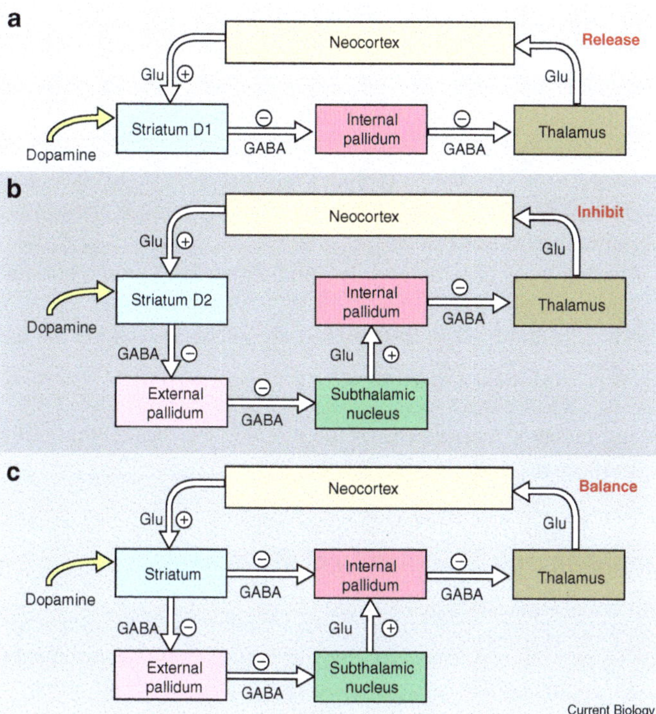

Fig. 6.2 Schematic diagrams of the basal ganglia circuits illustrating the direct pathway (**a**), indirect pathway (**b**), and their combined balanced activity (**c**). Panel (**a**) shows how dopaminergic activation of striatal D1 receptors facilitates the direct pathway, disinhibiting the thalamus and releasing cortical activity. Panel (**b**) shows how dopaminergic suppression of striatal D2 receptors modulates the indirect pathway through the external pallidum and subthalamic nucleus, ultimately increasing inhibition of the thalamus. Panel (**c**) illustrates the normal balance between these pathways, with glutamate (Glu) and GABA as the principal excitatory and inhibitory neurotransmitters, respectively

The Indirect Pathway: Inhibition of Movement

The indirect pathway inhibits voluntary movement by reducing excitatory output to the motor cortex. This pathway involves a more complex series of steps:

- The cortex stimulates the striatum, which inhibits the globus pallidus externus (GPe).
- Inhibition of GPe reduces its inhibitory effect on the subthalamic nucleus (STN).
- The disinhibited STN increases its excitatory output to the GPi.
- The GPi increases its inhibitory output to the thalamus, reducing thalamic stimulation of the motor cortex and suppressing movement.

Dopaminergic Modulation of Movement

Dopamine plays a crucial role in modulating basal ganglia activity. Dopamine is released by the substantia nigra pars compacta, and its effects differ between the direct and indirect pathways:

- *Direct Pathway:* Dopamine binds to D1 receptors on striatal neurons, facilitating the direct pathway and promoting movement.
- *Indirect Pathway:* Dopamine binds to D2 receptors on striatal neurons, inhibiting the indirect pathway and thus also promoting movement.

Basal Ganglia and Motor Control

The basal ganglia are essential for fine-tuning and regulating motor activity, ensuring that movements are smooth, coordinated, and contextually appropriate. Key motor functions include:

- *Motor Initiation*: Facilitating the initiation of voluntary movements by increasing motor cortical activity
- *Movement Coordination:* Coordinating the timing, force, and sequencing of muscle contractions
- *Motor Suppression:* Inhibiting unwanted movements or excessive muscle contractions to prevent involuntary or extraneous movements
- *Postural Control:* Contributing to the regulation of muscle tone and postural stability
- *Motor Learning:* Facilitating the learning of motor tasks and habits, as well as adapting motor responses to environmental changes

Detailed Neuroanatomical Organization

Striatal Architecture

The corpus striatum (caudate nucleus and putamen) consists of GABAergic neurons organized into two compartments: *striosomes* and *matrix*, which have different, though not yet fully understood, functions. The major projection neurons are type I and type II medium spiny neurons. Additionally, there are aspiny interneurons, including giant aspiny neurons that are cholinergic and medium aspiny neurons that are GABAergic.

- *Striosomes:* Receive input from the substantia nigra pars compacta, prefrontal cortex, and limbic regions; send output back to the SNc
- *Matrix:* Receives input from all cortical areas; sends output to the GPe, GPi, and SNr

Additional Basal Ganglia Structures

Lenticular Nucleus

An alternative anatomical grouping that includes the putamen, external medullary lamina, globus pallidus externus, internal medullary lamina, and globus pallidus internus.

Ventral Pallidum

The ventral pallidum is part of the globus pallidus located within the substantia innominata below the anterior commissure.

Nucleus Accumbens

The nucleus accumbens septi represents the ventral striatum at the junction of the caudate nucleus and putamen, containing GABAergic neurons. This structure is rich in opiate and dopamine receptors and is divided into:

- *Core:* Projects to the dorsolateral ventral pallidum
- *Shell:* Projects to the ventrolateral and ventromedial ventral striatum

Ventral Tegmental Area

The ventral tegmental area serves as the dopaminergic counterpart of the SNc for the limbic (ventral) striatum. This area is typically spared in Parkinson's disease, which explains why patients maintain intact reward-based dopaminergic functions while experiencing motor deficits.

Topographic Organization

Striatonigral fibers demonstrate precise topographic organization:

- Fibers from the head of the caudate project to the rostral third of the substantia nigra.
- Fibers from the dorsal putamen project to the lateral parts of the caudal two-thirds of the substantia nigra.
- Fibers from the ventral putamen project to the medial parts of the caudal two-thirds of the substantia nigra.

Functional Circuitry

Motor Circuit (Primary Motor Cortex)

This circuit is involved in voluntary movement control:

- Receives input from the primary motor cortex, supplementary motor area, and premotor cortex.
- Sends input to the ventral portions of the GPe (indirect pathway) and GPi (direct pathway).
- GPi neurons synapse on the ventral anterior (VA) and ventral lateral (VL) nuclei of the thalamus, with reciprocal feedback returning to the motor cortex.

Prefrontal Circuit

This circuit is involved in complex cognitive processes:

- Receives input from the dorsolateral prefrontal cortex
- Sends input to the dorsal portions of the GPe (indirect pathway) and GPi (direct pathway)
- Projects to the mediodorsal (MD) and ventral anterior (VA) thalamic nuclei

Limbic Circuit (Anterior Cingulate)

This circuit involves the ventral striatum (nucleus accumbens) and is involved in motivation; lesions result in apathy:

- Receives input from the anterior cingulate gyrus
- Sends output to the ventral parts of the GPe and GPi
- Projects to the mediodorsal (MD) thalamic nucleus, with additional outputs to the hypothalamus and ventral tegmental area

Major Fiber Pathways

Subthalamic Fasciculus

This bundle connects the globus pallidus to the subthalamus. It provides the excitatory input from the subthalamic nucleus to the GPi and also contains the reciprocal connections between the GPe and subthalamic nucleus.

Thalamic Fasciculus

This bundle connects the GPi to the thalamus and is formed from the junction of the lenticular fasciculus and ansa lenticularis. Technically, these fibers join to form the prerubral field (H field of Forel) before joining the thalamic fasciculus (H2 field of Forel). The thalamic fasciculus also contains cerebellothalamic fibers.

Lenticular Fasciculus

Also known as the H1 field of Forel, this pathway runs directly through the posterior limb of the internal capsule and between the subthalamus and zona incerta to reach the thalamus. It originates mostly from the medialmost layers of the GPi.

Ansa Lenticularis

This pathway runs anteriorly and loops around the medial edge of the internal capsule. It originates mostly from the lateralmost layers of the GPi.

Output Targets of the Basal Ganglia

The GPi provides inhibitory output to multiple targets:

- Thalamus (VA, VL, DM, CM, PF, and other nuclei).
- Habenula via pallidohabenular projections passing through the stria medullaris.
- Pedunculopontine nucleus (nucleus tegmenti pedunculopontis), which is important in the reticulospinal tract and represents the connection of the basal ganglia with the extrapyramidal system. The PPN is also a major component of the ascending reticular activating system.

Arterial Supply

Understanding the vascular supply to the basal ganglia is clinically important:

- Posterior cerebral artery penetrating branches supply the substantia nigra and subthalamic nucleus.
- Lateral striate arteries (lenticulostriate arteries) from the middle cerebral artery supply the striatum.
- Middle striate artery from the anterior cerebral artery supplies the head of the caudate.
- Anterior choroidal artery (from the internal carotid artery) provides branches to the globus pallidus.

Clinical Disorders of the Basal Ganglia

Dysfunction of the basal ganglia is associated with a variety of movement disorders that can be broadly classified as hypokinetic (decreased movement) or hyperkinetic (excessive involuntary movements).

Parkinson's Disease

Parkinson's disease results from the progressive degeneration of dopamine-producing neurons in the substantia nigra pars compacta, leading to an imbalance between the direct and indirect pathways. Destruction of the SNc decreases direct pathway activity and increases indirect pathway activity, both contributing to hypokinesia and rigidity. Saccadic eye movement abnormalities are also present due to abnormal coordination between the caudate nucleus, substantia nigra, and frontal eye fields.

Key Features:

- Methylphenyltetrahydropyridine (MPTP) is selectively toxic to dopaminergic neurons of the SNc.
- Electrical stimulation of the GP or STN can block the activity of these nuclei, suppressing Parkinsonian symptoms.

Cardinal Symptoms:

- Bradykinesia (slowness of movement)
- Resting tremor
- Rigidity
- Postural instability

Treatment Approaches:

- *Thalamotomy:* Stereotactic lesions to the VA and VL thalamic nuclei can suppress symptoms.
- *Pallidotomy:* Stereotactic lesions of the GPi or its output tracts can also suppress symptoms.
- *Deep Brain Stimulation:* Stimulation of the STN leads to disruption of the excitatory connections from the STN to the GPi, resulting in reduced GPi activity (similar mechanism to pallidotomy).

Huntington's Disease

Huntington's disease is an autosomal dominant genetic disorder characterized by progressive degeneration of the striatum, particularly the caudate nucleus and putamen. Destruction of the striatum leads to loss of inhibitory striatal input on both the GPi and GPe. This results in increased inhibition of the GPi by the GPe, leading to reduced GPi inhibition of the thalamus and thus increased thalamic firing. Consequently, the disorder is associated with hyperkinesia. Destruction of the head of the caudate leads to dementia because of the loss of prefrontal cortical control mechanisms mediated by the caudate.

Pathophysiology: D2 receptor-bearing neurons (enkephalinergic GABAergic neurons) are the first to degenerate, resulting in chorea. Later in the disease course, D1 receptor-bearing neurons (substance P-containing GABAergic neurons) degenerate, leading to athetosis and akinesias.

Clinical Features:

- Chorea (involuntary, jerky movements)
- Dystonia (muscle spasms and abnormal postures)
- Cognitive and psychiatric disturbances

Hemiballismus

Hemiballismus is characterized by wild and forceful hyperkinetic movements of the contralateral arms and legs. It results from destruction of the subthalamic nucleus, which leads to loss of excitatory input to the GPi. This causes decreased GPi inhibition of the thalamus and subsequent contralateral hyperkinesias.

Dystonia

Dystonia refers to a group of movement disorders characterized by sustained muscle contractions, resulting in abnormal postures or twisting movements. It can arise from basal ganglia dysfunction, particularly involving the putamen or globus pallidus.

Tardive Dyskinesia

Tardive dyskinesia results from long-term use of dopamine-blocking drugs, particularly antipsychotic medications. It leads to involuntary movements of the face, tongue, and limbs, and is thought to involve basal ganglia dysfunction related to dopamine receptor supersensitivity.

Tourette Syndrome

Tourette syndrome is a neuropsychiatric disorder characterized by motor and vocal tics (sudden, repetitive movements or vocalizations). It is thought to be related to dysfunction in basal ganglia circuits, particularly involving the striatum and thalamus.

Additional Movement Disorders

Sydenham's Chorea

A temporary post-streptococcal autoimmune disorder causing chorea, typically seen in children.

Choreoathetosis

A spectrum of hyperkinetic disorders caused by striatal degeneration, featuring characteristics of both chorea (brisk, graceful movements) and athetosis (slow, writhing movements of the extremities).

Dentatorubropallidoluysian Atrophy (DRPLA)

A trinucleotide repeat disorder affecting multiple structures including the dentate nucleus, red nucleus, globus pallidus, and subthalamic nucleus (Luys).

Toxin-Related Disorders

Methanol Toxicity

Methanol poisoning characteristically results in hemorrhage of the putamen due to selective vulnerability of this structure.

Carbon Monoxide Toxicity

Carbon monoxide poisoning results in hemorrhagic necrosis of the globus pallidus, reflecting the high metabolic demands and selective vulnerability of this structure to hypoxic injury.

Types of Abnormal Movements

- *Tremor at rest:* Rhythmic oscillations present when muscles are relaxed, characteristic of Parkinson's disease
- *Athetosis:* Slow, writhing movements of the extremities
- *Chorea:* Generalized brisk and graceful involuntary movements
- *Ballism:* Wild and forceful hyperkinetic movements of the arms and legs

Summary

The basal ganglia represent a complex network of subcortical nuclei that are essential for the regulation of movement, motor learning, and various cognitive functions. Understanding the anatomical organization, intricate circuitry involving direct and indirect pathways, and the critical role of dopaminergic modulation provides the foundation for comprehending the pathophysiology of movement disorders. The clinical manifestations of basal ganglia dysfunction range from the hypokinetic features of Parkinson's disease to the hyperkinetic movements seen in Huntington's disease and hemiballismus. Recognition of these disorders and their underlying neuroanatomical substrates is essential for medical students and residents to develop appropriate diagnostic and therapeutic strategies for patients with movement disorders.

The Cerebral Cortex

7

Introduction

The cerebral cortex, often referred to as the "gray matter" of the brain, constitutes the outermost layer of the cerebrum and represents the most highly evolved component of the human nervous system. This thin mantle of neural tissue, typically 2–4 mm in thickness, is responsible for the remarkable cognitive capabilities that distinguish humans from other species. Its grayish appearance derives primarily from the concentration of neuronal cell bodies, as opposed to the white matter beneath it, which consists predominantly of myelinated axons.

The cortex exhibits an intricate folded architecture that dramatically increases its surface area while maintaining a compact volume within the confines of the skull. This elaborate pattern of gyri (ridges) and sulci (valleys) allows the human brain to pack approximately 16 billion neurons into the cortical sheet. The folding pattern follows consistent anatomical landmarks that facilitate the identification of functionally specialized regions and provide a framework for clinical localization of lesions.

This chapter systematically examines the structural organization, functional specialization, and clinical significance of the cerebral cortex, providing the essential neuroanatomical foundation required for understanding both normal brain function and neurological disease.

V. Yanamadala, *Essential Neuroanatomy*,
https://doi.org/10.1007/978-3-032-26877-8_7

General Structure of the Cerebral Cortex

The cerebral cortex is divided into two hemispheres (left and right), each containing four major lobes that are delineated by prominent sulci and that subserve distinct functional roles in cognition and behavior.

Lobar Organization

The cerebral hemispheres are each subdivided into four principal lobes:

- *Frontal lobe*—occupies the anterior portion of the hemisphere, extending from the frontal pole to the central sulcus posteriorly and the lateral (Sylvian) fissure inferiorly
- *Parietal lobe*—lies posterior to the central sulcus and superior to the lateral fissure, extending to the parieto-occipital sulcus
- *Temporal lobe*—positions inferior to the lateral fissure and anterior to the occipital lobe
- *Occipital lobe*—forms the posterior pole of the hemisphere, separated from the parietal and temporal lobes by the parieto-occipital sulcus and the preoccipital notch

Each lobe is associated with specific functions related to sensory perception, motor control, language, memory, and higher-order cognitive processes. Understanding this lobar organization provides the foundation for clinical localization of lesions and interpretation of neurological deficits.

Cortical Cytoarchitecture and Laminar Organization

The cerebral cortex exhibits a highly organized laminar structure, typically consisting of six distinct layers arranged parallel to the cortical surface. This six-layered organization, termed neocortex or isocortex, characterizes most of the cortical mantle. The layers are conventionally numbered from I to VI, beginning at the pial surface and progressing toward the underlying white matter.

The Six Cortical Layers

Layer I (Molecular Layer)

The most superficial layer contains relatively few neuronal cell bodies, consisting primarily of apical dendrites from deeper pyramidal neurons, horizontal axons, and scattered Cajal-Retzius cells. This layer serves as a critical site for integrating information from multiple cortical sources.

Layer II (External Granular Layer)

Characterized by small, densely packed pyramidal and stellate neurons, this layer primarily sends projections to other cortical areas, contributing to cortico-cortical communication and information processing.

Layer III (External Pyramidal Layer)

Contains medium-sized pyramidal neurons that project to other cortical regions, playing essential roles in higher-order processing and inter-cortical communication. The size and density of pyramidal cells in this layer increase with cortical depth.

Layer IV (Internal Granular Layer)

The primary recipient of thalamic sensory input, particularly prominent in primary sensory cortices. This layer is especially well-developed in sensory areas, where it receives specific thalamocortical projections carrying sensory information. The termination of thalamic afferents in this layer is often visible as distinct bands called Baillarger's lines.

Layer V (Internal Pyramidal Layer)

Contains large pyramidal neurons, including the giant Betz cells in the primary motor cortex. These neurons give rise to major descending projection pathways to subcortical structures, including the corticospinal, corticobulbar, and corticostriatal tracts. This layer is particularly prominent in motor cortices.

Layer VI (Multiform Layer)

The deepest cortical layer sends reciprocal projections back to the thalamus, providing crucial feedback that modulates thalamocortical communication. This layer also contains diverse neuronal populations that contribute to local circuit processing.

Variations in Cortical Architecture

While the six-layered structure characterizes most cortex, significant regional variations exist:

Homotypic Cortex

Exhibits all six layers in their typical organization. This pattern predominates in association cortices, which integrate information from multiple sensory and motor systems.

Heterotypic Cortex

Displays modifications in which certain layers are either absent, merged, or particularly prominent. Two important subtypes include:

Granular Cortex—Characterized by prominent granular layers (II and IV) and reduced pyramidal cell layers. This pattern is typical of primary sensory cortices, which receive substantial thalamic input.

Agranular Cortex—Features prominent pyramidal cell layers with poorly developed or absent granular layers. This architecture characterizes primary motor cortex, reflecting its role in generating motor output rather than receiving sensory input.

Functional Organization of the Cerebral Cortex

The cerebral cortex exhibits remarkable functional specialization, with distinct regions dedicated to processing specific types of information or controlling particular functions. This specialization reflects both the intrinsic cytoarchitecture of cortical areas and their specific patterns of connectivity with subcortical structures and other cortical regions.

Primary Sensory Cortices

Primary sensory cortices serve as the initial cortical processing stations for sensory information. Each is organized topographically, meaning that adjacent regions of the sensory periphery map to adjacent cortical territories. This topographic organization allows for precise localization of sensory stimuli.

Primary Somatosensory Cortex

Located in the postcentral gyrus of the parietal lobe, immediately posterior to the central sulcus, the primary somatosensory cortex (S1) processes tactile sensations including touch, pressure, temperature, and proprioception. The cortical representation follows a somatotopic organization known as the sensory homunculus, in which body parts are mapped onto the cortical surface. Notably, areas with high sensory acuity (such as the hands, lips, and face) occupy disproportionately large cortical territories relative to their physical size, reflecting the principle of cortical magnification (Fig. 7.1).

The postcentral gyrus is subdivided into Brodmann areas 3a, 3b, 1, and 2, each receiving distinct types of sensory input. Areas 3b and 1 process cutaneous sensations, with rapidly adapting receptors projecting primarily to areas 1, 2, and 3b, while slowly adapting receptors target areas 1 and 3b. Area 3a receives input from muscle spindles, whereas areas 1 and 2 integrate information from joint receptors and deeper tissues. The termination of thalamocortical fibers in layer IV of S1 is visible histologically as the Band of Vicq-d'Azyr (Baillarger's lines).

Primary Visual Cortex

The primary visual cortex (V1, Brodmann area 17) occupies the banks of the calcarine sulcus in the medial occipital lobe, extending onto adjacent portions of the lingual gyrus inferiorly and the cuneus superiorly. This area receives direct input from the lateral

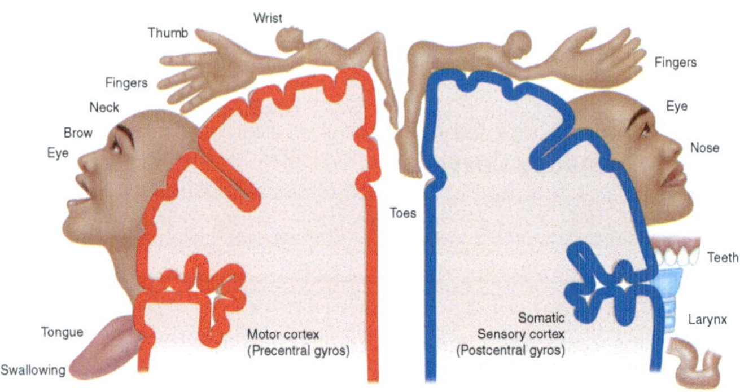

Fig. 7.1 Cortical homunculi illustrating the somatotopic organization of the primary motor cortex (precentral gyrus, red) and somatic sensory cortex (postcentral gyrus, blue). The disproportionate representation of the face, lips, tongue, hands, and fingers relative to the trunk and proximal limbs reflects the density of motor innervation and sensory receptor distribution across body regions

geniculate nucleus (LGN) of the thalamus via the optic radiations. The retinotopic organization of V1 preserves spatial relationships from the visual field, with the macula (central vision) represented in the posterior portion and peripheral vision mapped anteriorly.

A distinctive anatomical feature of V1 is the stria of Gennari, a heavily myelinated band of thalamocortical fibers terminating in layer IV that is visible to the naked eye in fresh specimens. V1 performs critical early processing of visual information, including the detection of edges, orientation, motion, and color. Visual information is then distributed to secondary visual cortices (areas 18 and 19) for higher-order processing.

Primary Auditory Cortex

The primary auditory cortex (A1, Brodmann areas 41 and 42) resides within the superior temporal gyrus, specifically on Heschl's gyrus (transverse temporal gyri), which lies within the lateral (Sylvian) fissure. This region receives tonotopically organized input from the medial geniculate nucleus of the thalamus, with different frequencies of sound mapped systematically across the cortical surface. The primary auditory cortex performs initial processing of sound features, including frequency, intensity, and temporal patterns.

Primary Gustatory Cortex

Taste information is processed in the primary gustatory cortex, which is located in the anterior insula and the frontal operculum (part of the inferior frontal gyrus). This region receives input from the ventral posteromedial nucleus of the thalamus and integrates gustatory information with olfactory and visceral sensations.

Primary Olfactory Cortex

Unlike other sensory modalities, olfactory information bypasses the thalamus and projects directly to primary olfactory cortex, which includes the piriform cortex and the olfactory tubercle in the temporal lobe. These paleocortical structures, evolutionarily older than the six-layered neocortex, receive direct input from the olfactory bulb via the olfactory tract.

Motor Cortices

The motor cortices orchestrate voluntary movement through a hierarchical organization that includes primary motor areas for execution and secondary areas for planning and coordination.

Primary Motor Cortex

The primary motor cortex (M1, Brodmann area 4) occupies the posterior portion of the precentral gyrus in the frontal lobe, immediately anterior to the central sulcus. This region exhibits an agranular architecture with a prominent layer V containing giant Betz cells, whose axons contribute to the corticospinal tract. Like the somatosensory cortex, M1 is organized somatotopically as a motor homunculus, with body parts requiring fine motor control (hands, face, tongue) represented by disproportionately large cortical areas.

Motor commands generated in M1 descend primarily through the corticospinal and corticobulbar tracts to activate lower motor neurons in the spinal cord and brainstem. The motor output is predominantly contralateral, meaning that the left motor cortex controls the right side of the body and vice versa.

Premotor Cortex

The premotor cortex (Brodmann area 6) lies immediately anterior to M1 in the anterior portion of the precentral gyrus. This region participates in motor planning, coordination of complex movements, and integration of sensory information to guide motor actions. The premotor cortex is particularly active during the preparation phase of voluntary movements and plays a crucial role in motor learning and the formation of motor programs.

Supplementary Motor Area

The supplementary motor area (SMA, part of area 6) occupies the medial surface of the superior frontal gyrus, extending onto the medial wall of the hemisphere. This region is essential for the planning and sequencing of complex, internally generated movements, particularly those requiring bilateral coordination. The SMA becomes activated well before movement execution, suggesting its role in motor preparation and intention.

Frontal Eye Fields

The frontal eye fields (Brodmann area 8) are located in the posterior part of the middle frontal gyrus, anterior to the premotor cortex. These regions control voluntary saccadic eye movements and are critical for directing visual attention to relevant stimuli in the environment.

Association Cortices

Association cortices comprise the majority of the human cortical surface and serve to integrate information from multiple sensory modalities and motor systems, enabling complex cognitive functions including language, spatial reasoning, decision-making, and abstract thought. These regions do not directly process sensory input or generate motor output but instead synthesize information for higher-order processing.

Prefrontal Cortex

The prefrontal cortex occupies the anterior portion of the frontal lobe (Brodmann areas 9–12, 46, 47) and represents the pinnacle of cortical evolution. This expansive region subserves executive functions including working memory, attention, planning, decision-making, behavioral inhibition, and cognitive flexibility. The prefrontal cortex integrates information from diverse sources to guide goal-directed behavior and is critical for personality, social cognition, and emotional regulation.

The prefrontal cortex can be subdivided into functionally distinct regions:

Dorsolateral Prefrontal Cortex (DLPFC)—mediates cognitive control, working memory maintenance, attention, and organization of complex thoughts and behaviors.

Ventromedial Prefrontal Cortex (VMPFC)—essential for emotional regulation, social behavior, moral reasoning, and value-based decision-making. This region integrates visceral and emotional signals into the decision-making process.

Orbitofrontal Cortex (OFC)—processes reward and punishment signals, evaluates expected outcomes, and regulates social behavior and emotional responses. Dysfunction in this area results in impulsivity and socially inappropriate behavior.

Parietal Association Cortex

The posterior parietal cortex (Brodmann areas 5, 7, 39, 40) integrates somatosensory, visual, and auditory information to construct a coherent representation of space and body position. This region is critical for visuospatial processing, attention, and the integration of sensory information with motor planning. The inferior parietal lobule, including the supramarginal gyrus (area 40) and angular gyrus (area 39), plays essential roles in language, mathematical processing, and spatial cognition.

Lesions of the right posterior parietal cortex frequently result in hemispatial neglect syndrome, a striking disorder in which patients fail to attend to or acknowledge stimuli in the left half of space. Left parietal lesions can produce apraxias (impaired execution of learned movements) and Gerstmann syndrome (agraphia, acalculia, finger agnosia, and left-right disorientation).

Temporal Association Cortex

The lateral temporal cortex (areas 20, 21, 22, 37) performs high-level processing of auditory information, including language comprehension, object recognition, and semantic memory. The superior and middle temporal gyri contain regions essential for complex auditory processing, while the inferior temporal cortex is specialized for visual object recognition. The temporo-parietal-occipital junction integrates information from multiple sensory modalities to support complex cognitive functions.

Language Centers

Language processing relies on a distributed network of cortical regions predominantly lateralized to the left hemisphere in most individuals (approximately 95% of right-handed and 70% of left-handed individuals). The two classical language areas are Broca's and Wernicke's areas.

Broca's Area

Broca's area (Brodmann areas 44 and 45) is located in the posterior portion of the inferior frontal gyrus in the left frontal lobe. This region is crucial for speech production, grammatical processing, and the motor aspects of language. Damage to Broca's area results in Broca's aphasia (expressive or motor aphasia), characterized by non-fluent, effortful speech with relatively preserved comprehension. Patients with Broca's aphasia produce short, telegraphic utterances with simplified grammar but generally understand spoken language.

The Wada test, in which one hemisphere is temporarily anesthetized through intracarotid injection of sodium amobarbital, can be performed pre-surgically to determine the lateralization of language function and help prevent post-operative language deficits.

Wernicke's Area

Wernicke's area is situated in the posterior portion of the superior temporal gyrus (Brodmann area 22) in the left hemisphere. This region is essential for language comprehension and the semantic processing of spoken and written language. Lesions of Wernicke's area produce Wernicke's aphasia (receptive or sensory aphasia), characterized by fluent but often meaningless speech accompanied by severe impairment in comprehension. Patients may produce well-articulated sentences that lack semantic content (jargon aphasia) and fail to recognize their linguistic errors.

Broca's and Wernicke's areas are interconnected by the arcuate fasciculus, a white matter tract that enables the integration of language production and comprehension. Damage to this connection results in conduction aphasia, in which patients retain fluent speech and comprehension but demonstrate severe impairment in repetition.

Brodmann's Cytoarchitectonic Map and Functional Correlates

Korbinian Brodmann's seminal work in the early twentieth century identified 52 distinct cortical regions based on cytoarchitectonic differences in cellular organization, cell types, and laminar structure. Although modern neuroimaging and molecular techniques have revealed additional functional subdivisions, Brodmann's numerical system remains the standard nomenclature for cortical areas in clinical and research settings. The following section details the major functional correlates of Brodmann areas relevant to clinical practice (Fig. 7.2).

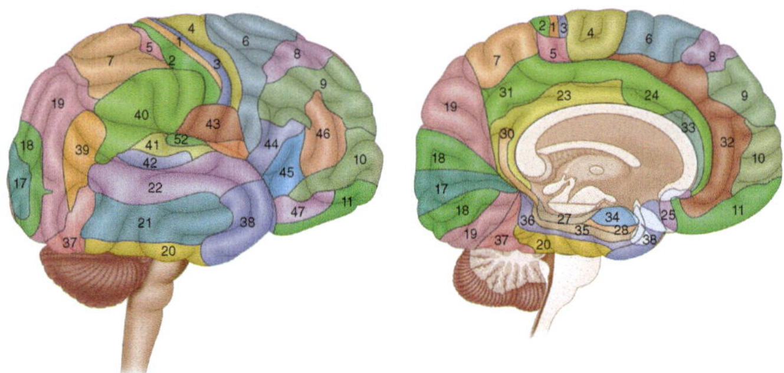

Fig. 7.2 Brodmann areas of the cerebral cortex shown on lateral (left) and medial (right) views of the left hemisphere. Each color-coded region represents a cytoarchitecturally distinct cortical area as defined by Brodmann's 1909 parcellation scheme, numbered according to the original classification. Key areas visible on the lateral surface include the primary motor cortex (area 4), premotor and supplementary motor cortex (area 6), prefrontal cortex (areas 9, 10, 11, 46, 47), primary somatosensory cortex (areas 1, 2, 3), somatosensory association cortex (areas 5, 7), primary auditory cortex (areas 41, 42), auditory association cortex (area 22), Broca's speech area (areas 44, 45), primary visual cortex (area 17), visual association cortex (areas 18, 19), and inferotemporal and fusiform regions (areas 20, 21, 37, 38). The medial surface additionally reveals the anterior cingulate cortex (areas 24, 25), posterior cingulate cortex (areas 23, 31), retrosplenial cortex (areas 29, 30), precuneus (area 7/31), and medial prefrontal and orbitofrontal regions (areas 10, 11, 12, 25, 32). Area 52 (parainsular cortex) is visible at the depth of the lateral sulcus on the lateral view. The Brodmann map remains the standard reference system for localizing functional neuroimaging findings and defining cortical lesion topography in clinical neuroscience

Somatosensory and Motor Areas

Areas 1, 2, 3a, 3b (Primary Somatosensory Cortex)

Located in the postcentral gyrus, these areas process distinct aspects of somatosensory information. Rapidly adapting skin receptors project to areas 1, 2, and 3b; slowly adapting receptors to areas 1 and 3b; joint receptors to areas 1 and 2; muscle spindle receptors to area 3a; and receptors in deep tissues to areas 1 and 2. The Band of Vicq-d'Azyr marks the termination of thalamocortical fibers in layer IV of these regions.

Area 4 (Primary Motor Cortex)
Occupies the posterior precentral gyrus and generates voluntary motor commands that descend via the corticospinal and corticobulbar tracts.

Area 6 (Premotor and Supplementary Motor Cortex)
The anterior precentral gyrus contains premotor cortex involved in motor planning and coordination.

Area 8 (Frontal Eye Fields)
Located anterior to area 6, this region controls voluntary saccadic eye movements and visual attention.

Visual and Visuospatial Areas

Area 17 (Primary Visual Cortex, V1)
The calcarine cortex, including the upper lingual gyrus and lower cuneus, processes basic visual features. The stria of Gennari marks thalamocortical fiber terminations from the lateral geniculate nucleus in layer IV.

Areas 18, 19 (Secondary Visual Cortex)
The remaining occipital lobe processes higher-order visual features including form, motion, and complex patterns. Area 19 contains the occipital eye fields, involved in object-oriented movement, particularly smooth pursuit.

Areas 5, 7 (Tertiary Sensory Cortex)
Located in the superior parietal lobule above the supramarginal gyrus, these association areas integrate visual and somatosensory information for spatial processing. Lesions produce contralateral neglect syndrome, particularly when involving the right hemisphere.

Somatosensory Association Areas

Area 40 (Secondary Somatosensory Cortex)
The supramarginal gyrus, located just posterior to the postcentral gyrus, integrates somatosensory information and participates in language and spatial processing.

Auditory and Language Areas

Areas 41, 42 (Primary Auditory Cortex)
The superior temporal gyrus, particularly Heschl's gyrus (area 41, the transverse temporal gyri), processes basic auditory features including frequency, intensity, and temporal patterns.

Area 22 (Secondary Auditory Cortex, Wernicke's Area)
The superior and middle temporal gyri process complex auditory information. The posterior superior temporal gyrus constitutes Wernicke's area; lesions result in sensory (receptive) aphasia with impaired language comprehension despite fluent speech production.

Areas 44, 45 (Broca's Area)
The frontal operculum (area 44) and triangular part of the inferior frontal gyrus (area 45) control speech production. Lesions produce motor (expressive) aphasia characterized by non-fluent, effortful speech with preserved comprehension.

Prefrontal and Executive Areas

Areas 9, 10, 11, 12 (Prefrontal Cortex)
The orbital gyri, gyrus rectus, and anterior portions of the superior and middle frontal gyri mediate executive functions, including personality, motivation, planning, judgment, and decision-making.

Parietal Association Areas

Areas 39, 40 (Parietal Association Cortex)
The angular gyrus (39) and supramarginal gyrus (40) integrate multimodal sensory information. Right-sided lesions frequently produce neglect syndromes, while left-sided lesions can cause apraxia, alexia, and other disconnection syndromes.

Hemispheric Lateralization and Functional Asymmetry

Although the two cerebral hemispheres appear structurally symmetric, they exhibit profound functional asymmetries. This lateralization of function reflects specialized processing capabilities that develop through a combination of genetic programming and environmental influences.

Left Hemisphere Dominance

The left hemisphere typically dominates language functions, analytical reasoning, mathematical processing, and sequential information processing. Broca's and Wernicke's areas are overwhelmingly lateralized to the left hemisphere, particularly in right-handed individuals. The left hemisphere excels at processing temporal sequences, logical analysis, and verbal memory.

Right Hemisphere Specialization

The right hemisphere specializes in visuospatial processing, facial recognition, emotional prosody, artistic abilities, and holistic information processing. It is dominant for spatial attention, body schema representation, and the recognition of familiar faces. The right hemisphere also plays a critical role in processing emotional content, including the interpretation of facial expressions and emotional tone of speech (emotional prosody).

Clinical evaluation of hemispheric specialization reveals that right hemisphere lesions often produce deficits in spatial awareness (neglect), prosody (monotone speech), and emotional processing, while left hemisphere lesions typically cause language impairments (aphasias) and deficits in analytical reasoning.

Cortical Plasticity and Reorganization

The cerebral cortex demonstrates remarkable plasticity—the ability to reorganize structure and function in response to experience, learning, or injury. This adaptive capacity underlies skill acquisition, memory formation, and recovery from brain damage.

Cortical plasticity is most prominent during critical periods of development when neural circuits are particularly sensitive to environmental input. The developing brain can compensate for injuries far more effectively than the mature brain, sometimes transferring functions from damaged regions to intact areas. For example, children who undergo hemispherectomy for intractable epilepsy can develop remarkably normal language function if the surgery occurs before adolescence.

Even in adults, the cortex retains significant plasticity. Learning new skills produces measurable changes in cortical representation, with practice leading to expansion of relevant cortical territories. Following stroke or traumatic injury, intensive rehabilitation can promote functional recovery through reorganization of perilesional cortex and recruitment of alternative networks. Understanding cortical plasticity has transformed approaches to neurorehabilitation and informed strategies for optimizing recovery after brain injury.

The Frontal Lobe: Detailed Anatomy and Function

The frontal lobe, the largest of the four cerebral lobes, occupies approximately one-third of the cerebral cortex and serves as the command center for voluntary movement, executive function, personality, and speech production. Its extensive connections with other cortical and subcortical structures enable integration of sensory information, emotional states, and motivational drives into coherent goal-directed behavior.

Anatomical Boundaries and Subdivisions

The frontal lobe extends from the frontal pole anteriorly to the central sulcus posteriorly, which separates it from the parietal lobe. Its inferior boundary is demarcated by the lateral (Sylvian) fissure, which separates it from the temporal lobe. On the medial surface, the cingulate sulcus defines its inferior extent. The frontal lobe can be subdivided into several functionally distinct regions based on cytoarchitecture and connectivity patterns.

Prefrontal Cortex

The prefrontal cortex comprises the anterior frontal lobe and orchestrates the highest levels of cognitive function. The dorsolateral prefrontal cortex (DLPFC) governs working memory, cognitive control, attention, and executive planning. The ventromedial prefrontal cortex (VMPFC) integrates emotional information into decision-making and regulates social behavior. The orbitofrontal cortex (OFC), located above the orbits, evaluates reward and punishment, enabling adaptive decision-making in uncertain environments.

Motor and Premotor Cortices

The primary motor cortex (M1, area 4) occupies the posterior precentral gyrus and directly controls voluntary movements through its projections to the spinal cord and brainstem. The premotor cortex (area 6) lies anteriorly and participates in movement planning and coordination. The supplementary motor area (SMA), on the medial surface, sequences complex movements and coordinates bilateral actions.

Speech Production Centers

Broca's area (areas 44 and 45) in the left inferior frontal gyrus controls the motor aspects of speech production and grammatical processing, making it essential for fluent, articulate speech.

Anterior Cingulate Cortex

The anterior cingulate cortex (ACC) on the medial surface integrates cognitive and emotional processing, monitors conflicts and errors, and regulates attention and motivation. The ACC plays crucial roles in pain processing, emotional regulation, and cognitive control. Stereotactic radiofrequency ablation of the anterior cingulate (anterior cingulotomy) is sometimes employed as a treatment for refractory obsessive-compulsive disorder.

Major White Matter Connections

The frontal lobe maintains extensive connections with other brain regions through several major white matter pathways. The corticospinal and corticobulbar tracts convey motor commands from M1 to lower motor neurons. Thalamocortical and corticothalamic connections mediate bidirectional communication with the thalamus. Extensive reciprocal connections with limbic structures (amygdala, hippocampus) integrate emotional information into decision-making and behavioral control. Corticostriatal projections to the basal ganglia participate in feedback loops that modulate motor control and habit formation.

Clinical Syndromes of Frontal Lobe Damage

Frontal lobe lesions produce diverse neurological and neuropsychiatric manifestations depending on the specific region affected.

Motor Deficits

Lesions of the primary motor cortex cause contralateral weakness or paralysis (hemiparesis or hemiplegia). Damage to premotor or supplementary motor areas impairs the planning and sequencing of complex movements while preserving basic motor strength.

Executive Dysfunction

Dorsolateral prefrontal lesions produce executive dysfunction characterized by impaired working memory, reduced cognitive flexibility, poor planning, and difficulty with complex problem-solving. Patients may perseverate on tasks, struggle with abstract reasoning, and exhibit deficits in attention and concentration.

Behavioral and Personality Changes

Ventromedial and orbitofrontal lesions lead to dramatic personality changes, including impulsivity, poor judgment, social inappropriateness, emotional lability, and reduced insight. The classic case of Phineas Gage, who sustained frontal lobe damage in a railroad accident, exemplifies these changes. Patients may display disinhibited behavior, lack of empathy, and inability to learn from negative consequences—a constellation termed frontal lobe syndrome.

Language Disorders

Left frontal lesions affecting Broca's area produce expressive aphasia with non-fluent, effortful speech but relatively preserved comprehension. Right frontal lesions can impair motor prosody, resulting in monotone speech that lacks normal emotional inflection.

Frontal Eye Field Lesions

Acute lesions of the frontal eye fields produce an inability to voluntarily direct gaze toward the contralateral side, with eyes deviating toward the side of the lesion ("looking toward the lesion").

The Parietal Lobe: Sensory Integration and Spatial Processing

The parietal lobe lies posterior to the central sulcus and superior to the lateral fissure, extending posteriorly to the parieto-occipital sulcus. This region integrates somatosensory information with visual, auditory, and motor data to construct coherent representations of body position, spatial relationships, and the locations of objects in extrapersonal space.

Anatomical Subdivisions

The parietal lobe is divided by the postcentral sulcus into anterior and posterior regions. The postcentral gyrus contains the primary somatosensory cortex (Brodmann areas 3a, 3b, 1, 2), while posterior parietal regions (areas 5, 7, 39, 40) serve associative functions. The intraparietal sulcus separates the superior and inferior parietal lobules, which have distinct functional specializations.

The superior parietal lobule processes spatial information for reaching and grasping movements, integrating visual and proprioceptive signals to guide motor actions. The inferior parietal lobule comprises the supramarginal gyrus (area 40) and angular gyrus (area 39), which participate in language, reading, writing, mathematical reasoning, and complex sensorimotor integration.

Functional Specializations

The parietal lobe serves as a critical hub for multisensory integration, constructing unified representations of space, body, and objects from diverse sensory streams. The posterior parietal cortex transforms sensory information into motor coordinates for action, enabling visually guided reaching, grasping, and manipulation of objects. This sensorimotor transformation allows us to interact seamlessly with the environment.

The left inferior parietal lobule participates in language networks, particularly in phonological processing, reading, and writing. The angular gyrus is essential for mapping visual word forms onto their semantic representations during reading. Damage to this region can produce alexia with agraphia (inability to read or write despite intact speech).

Clinical Syndromes

Right parietal lesions characteristically produce hemispatial neglect, a dramatic syndrome in which patients fail to attend to, respond to, or report stimuli in the left half of space despite intact primary sensory function. Patients may eat food only from the right side of their plate, dress only the right side of their body, and deny ownership of their left limbs. This reflects a disruption in spatial attention and body representation rather than a primary sensory deficit.

Left parietal lesions produce a distinct constellation of deficits. Apraxias result from damage to regions that store motor programs for learned, skilled movements. Patients can understand commands and have adequate motor strength but cannot correctly execute familiar actions like using tools or making gestures. Ideomotor apraxia affects pantomimed actions, while ideational apraxia impairs the sequencing of multi-step actions.

Gerstmann syndrome, resulting from left angular gyrus lesions, comprises four cardinal features: agraphia (impaired writing), acalculia (impaired calculation), finger agnosia (inability to identify fingers), and left-right disorientation. This tetrad suggests a fundamental deficit in symbolic representation and spatial reasoning. Bilateral parietal damage can produce Balint syndrome, characterized by simultanagnosia (inability to perceive the visual field as a whole), optic ataxia (impaired visually guided reaching), and oculomotor apraxia (difficulty directing gaze voluntarily).

The Occipital Lobe: Visual Processing and Perception

The occipital lobe, occupying the posterior pole of the cerebral hemisphere, is dedicated almost exclusively to visual processing. Despite representing the smallest of the four major lobes, it contains the most sophisticated neural machinery for analyzing visual information, transforming patterns of light detected by the retina into our rich, multifaceted visual experience of the world.

Anatomical Organization

The occipital lobe is bounded anteriorly by the parieto-occipital sulcus on the medial surface and by an imaginary line connecting the parieto-occipital sulcus to the preoccipital notch on the lateral surface. The medial surface is divided by the calcarine sulcus into the cuneus superiorly and the lingual gyrus inferiorly. The lateral occipital gyri extend over the lateral convexity.

The calcarine sulcus is particularly significant because it contains the primary visual cortex (V1, Brodmann area 17), also known as the striate cortex due to the prominent stria of Gennari visible in layer IV. This distinctive myelinated band represents the termination of thalamocortical fibers from the lateral geniculate nucleus, marking the entry point for visual information into the cortex.

Retinotopic Organization and Visual Field Representation

The primary visual cortex maintains a precise retinotopic map of the visual field, with adjacent points in visual space represented by adjacent cortical neurons. This topographic organization preserves spatial relationships throughout the visual pathways from retina to cortex. The fovea, responsible for high-acuity central vision, occupies a disproportionately large representation in the posterior occipital pole, reflecting the principle of cortical magnification.

Visual field representation in the calcarine cortex follows specific anatomical principles. The upper visual field projects to the inferior bank of the calcarine sulcus (lingual gyrus), while the lower visual field maps to the superior bank (cuneus). The central visual field occupies posterior cortex near the occipital pole, whereas peripheral vision is represented more anteriorly. This organization has important clinical implications: lesions of the superior calcarine cortex produce inferior visual field defects (inferior quadrantanopia), while inferior calcarine lesions cause superior field defects.

Hierarchical Visual Processing

Visual processing proceeds through a hierarchical series of cortical areas, each extracting increasingly complex features from the visual input. V1 neurons respond to simple features such as oriented edges, motion direction, and color. This information is then distributed to secondary visual areas (V2, V3, V4, V5/MT) surrounding V1, which analyze more complex features. V2 processes contours and surfaces, V3 contributes to form perception, V4 specializes in color processing, and V5/MT in the superior temporal sulcus analyzes motion.

Beyond these early visual areas, visual information flows into two major processing streams. The dorsal stream projects from occipital cortex through posterior parietal regions, processing spatial information and visual guidance of action (the 'where' or 'how' pathway). The ventral stream projects to inferior temporal cortex, specializing in object identification and recognition (the 'what' pathway). This dual-stream organization reflects the fundamental distinction between perceiving object identity versus spatial location and action guidance.

Clinical Syndromes of Occipital Lobe Damage

Visual Field Defects

Lesions of the primary visual cortex produce characteristic visual field defects. Unilateral occipital damage causes homonymous hemianopia—loss of vision in the contralateral visual field of both eyes. The presence of macular sparing (preservation of central vision) often indicates cortical rather than subcortical lesions, as the macular representation in posterior occipital cortex receives dual vascular supply from both posterior cerebral and middle cerebral arteries.

Quadrantanopias result from partial occipital lesions affecting either the superior or inferior visual cortex. Bilateral occipital damage can produce cortical blindness, in which patients lose all conscious vision despite intact pupillary reflexes. Some patients with cortical blindness develop Anton syndrome, a remarkable condition in which they deny their blindness and may confabulate visual experiences.

Visual Agnosias

Damage to visual association areas can produce visual agnosias—disorders of visual recognition despite adequate elementary vision. Apperceptive agnosia results from lesions of early visual association cortex and impairs the ability to perceive object shape and form. Patients cannot copy or match simple figures. Associative agnosia, caused by more anterior ventral stream lesions, preserves perception but disrupts the connection between visual percepts and stored semantic knowledge. Patients can copy drawings they cannot identify.

Prosopagnosia, or face blindness, typically results from bilateral lesions of the fusiform gyri in the ventral occipitotemporal region. Patients lose the ability to recognize familiar faces, including their own reflection, though they may recognize individuals by voice or other cues. This striking disorder demonstrates the existence of face-selective neural mechanisms in the ventral visual stream.

Achromatopsia and Motion Blindness

Cerebral achromatopsia results from damage to area V4 in the ventral occipitotemporal cortex. Patients perceive the world in shades of gray despite intact retinal color vision. This disorder demonstrates that color perception depends on cortical processing beyond the retina. Conversely, selective damage to area V5/MT can produce akinetopsia or motion blindness, in which patients cannot perceive visual motion. Moving objects appear as a series of static images, making tasks like crossing streets extremely difficult.

Complex Visual Phenomena

Occipital lobe lesions can produce various positive visual phenomena. Visual hallucinations may arise from irritative lesions or seizures, typically consisting of simple, unformed images (photopsias, phosphenes) with occipital cortex involvement. Charles Bonnet syndrome describes complex visual hallucinations in patients with vision loss, thought to result from spontaneous activity in deafferented visual cortex. Palinopsia, the persistence or recurrence of visual images after the stimulus has been removed, can occur with posterior cerebral lesions.

The Temporal Lobe: Memory, Language, and Emotion

The temporal lobe, situated inferior to the lateral fissure and anterior to the occipital lobe, performs critical functions in auditory processing, language comprehension, object recognition, memory formation, and emotional processing. Its diverse functions reflect the heterogeneity of its constituent structures, which include primary sensory cortex, multimodal association areas, and limbic structures essential for memory and emotion.

Gross Anatomical Organization

The lateral surface of the temporal lobe is organized into three parallel gyri:

Superior Temporal Gyrus

Contains the primary auditory cortex (Heschl's gyrus) on its superior surface within the Sylvian fissure. The posterior portion includes Wernicke's area, essential for language comprehension. The superior temporal sulcus on its inferior border marks the boundary with the middle temporal gyrus.

Middle Temporal Gyrus
Participates in word retrieval, sentence processing during language comprehension, and integration of auditory and visual information for object and face recognition.

Inferior Temporal Gyrus
Specialized for high-level visual object recognition and face processing. The fusiform face area (FFA) within this region is selectively activated by face stimuli; damage produces prosopagnosia, an inability to recognize familiar faces despite intact object recognition.

Additional Temporal Lobe Structures

The inferior surface contains the occipitotemporal gyrus (fusiform gyrus), parahippocampal gyrus, and lingual gyrus. The medial temporal lobe houses critical limbic structures, including the hippocampus, amygdala, and entorhinal cortex, which collectively orchestrate memory formation and emotional processing.

Functional Domains of the Temporal Lobe

Auditory Processing
The primary auditory cortex receives tonotopically organized projections from the medial geniculate nucleus and performs initial cortical processing of sound. The surrounding auditory association cortex analyzes complex auditory patterns, enabling recognition of speech, music, and environmental sounds. The superior temporal sulcus is particularly important for processing socially relevant auditory information such as vocal emotional expressions.

Language Comprehension
Wernicke's area in the posterior superior temporal gyrus is essential for understanding spoken and written language. This region maps sounds onto meanings and accesses semantic knowledge.

Damage produces Wernicke's aphasia, characterized by fluent but meaningless speech (semantic paraphasias) and severely impaired comprehension. The angular gyrus at the temporo-parietal junction contributes to reading, writing, and mathematical processing.

Memory Formation and Consolidation

The hippocampus in the medial temporal lobe is indispensable for forming new declarative memories (episodic and semantic). It binds together distributed cortical representations to create coherent memory traces and supports spatial navigation through place cells that encode location. The adjacent entorhinal cortex serves as the primary gateway for cortical information entering the hippocampus. Bilateral hippocampal damage produces profound anterograde amnesia, as famously demonstrated by patient H.M., who could no longer form new long-term memories after bilateral medial temporal lobectomy.

The perirhinal and parahippocampal cortices contribute to recognition memory and contextual memory, respectively. Together, these medial temporal structures form a critical memory system that has been extensively studied in neurodegenerative diseases such as Alzheimer's disease, which characteristically affects the entorhinal cortex and hippocampus in its earliest stages.

Emotional Processing

The amygdala, an almond-shaped nuclear complex in the anterior medial temporal lobe, processes the emotional significance of stimuli, particularly those related to threat and fear. It receives highly processed sensory information and projects to hypothalamic and brainstem autonomic centers, enabling rapid emotional responses. The amygdala is essential for emotional learning, fear conditioning, and modulation of memory consolidation based on emotional significance.

The temporal pole at the anterior tip of the temporal lobe integrates social and emotional information, contributing to social cognition, theory of mind, and the recognition of emotional expressions.

Clinical Syndromes of Temporal Lobe Pathology

Memory Disorders

Bilateral medial temporal damage produces severe anterograde amnesia with inability to form new declarative memories. Alzheimer's disease characteristically begins with hippocampal and entorhinal degeneration, producing progressive memory decline. Korsakoff syndrome, often resulting from thiamine deficiency in chronic alcoholism, damages the mammillary bodies and medial thalamus, producing both anterograde and retrograde amnesia along with confabulation.

Aphasias

Left temporal lesions produce various language disorders. Wernicke's aphasia results from posterior superior temporal damage, while transcortical sensory aphasia results from lesions that isolate Wernicke's area from other language zones. Primary progressive aphasia, often associated with frontotemporal dementia, produces gradual language deterioration beginning with word-finding difficulties.

Temporal Lobe Epilepsy

The medial temporal lobe, particularly the hippocampus and amygdala, is a common focus for seizure activity. Complex partial seizures originating from these structures produce alterations in consciousness, automatisms, experiential phenomena (déjà vu, jamais vu), and autonomic symptoms. Chronic temporal lobe epilepsy can lead to hippocampal sclerosis and progressive memory decline.

Visual Recognition Disorders

Lesions of the inferior temporal cortex produce visual agnosias—the inability to recognize objects despite intact elementary vision. Prosopagnosia (face blindness) results from damage to the fusiform face area, while other forms of visual agnosia affect object recognition more generally.

Auditory Hallucinations

Abnormal temporal lobe activity, particularly in auditory cortex and association areas, can produce auditory hallucinations. These are common in schizophrenia and can also occur in temporal lobe epilepsy and some neurodegenerative diseases.

Emotional Dysregulation

Bilateral medial temporal damage, particularly involving the amygdala, produces Klüver-Bucy syndrome, characterized by hyperorality, hypersexuality, visual agnosia, placidity, and loss of fear responses. Less extensive amygdalar damage can result in altered emotional processing, anxiety disorders, or inappropriate social behavior.

The Limbic System: Emotion, Memory, and Motivated Behavior

The limbic system comprises a collection of interconnected structures that form a ring around the brainstem and corpus callosum. Originally conceived as the neural substrate for emotion, the limbic system is now recognized as a complex network essential for emotional processing, memory formation, motivation, and the integration of visceral and emotional states with cognition and behavior. All limbic structures uniquely express the cell surface glycoprotein known as limbic system-associated membrane protein (LAMP), which serves as a molecular marker for this functional system.

Principal Components of the Limbic System

Cingulate Gyrus

The cingulate gyrus is a curved convolution that arches over the corpus callosum, representing transitional cortex (mesocortex or juxtallocortex) between the six-layered neocortex and the phylogenetically older allocortex. The anterior cingulate cortex subserves attention, conflict monitoring, error detection, and emotional regulation. As noted previously, anterior cingulotomy using stereotactic radiofrequency ablation can be employed as a treatment for refractory obsessive-compulsive disorder. The dorsal and posterior cingulate regions contribute to decision-making and self-referential processing. The isthmus of the cingulate gyrus forms a bridge connecting the cingulate and parahippocampal gyri.

Parahippocampal Gyrus

This medial temporal structure surrounds the hippocampus and contains several functionally specialized regions. The entorhinal cortex serves as the primary interface between the hippocampus and neocortex, receiving convergent input from the cingulate gyrus, olfactory bulb, basolateral amygdala, prelimbic cortex (Brodmann area 32), and sensory association cortices processing visual, auditory, and gustatory information. The entorhinal cortex is one of the earliest sites affected by Alzheimer's pathology. The piriform cortex represents paleocortex specialized for olfactory processing. The uncus forms the anterior hook of the parahippocampal gyrus and contains portions of the amygdala and entorhinal cortex.

The parahippocampal gyrus is separated from the rest of the temporal lobe by the collateral sulcus laterally and the rhinal sulcus more anteriorly. The hippocampus lies deep within the parahippocampal gyrus, forming a prominence in the floor of the inferior horn of the lateral ventricle called the calcar avis.

Hippocampus

The hippocampus represents archicortex, an evolutionarily ancient three-layered cortical structure critical for memory consolidation and spatial navigation. Anatomically, the hippocampus is subdivided along its long axis into the pes (foot), head, body, and tail. The hippocampal formation includes the dentate gyrus, hippocampus proper (with subfields CA1-CA4), and subiculum.

The hippocampus serves as the gateway for transferring information from short-term to long-term memory storage, particularly for declarative (explicit) memories of facts and events.

Spatial memory depends critically on hippocampal place cells that encode specific locations. The hippocampus projects via the fornix to the mammillary bodies, anterior thalamus, and septal nuclei, forming key components of the classical Papez circuit for emotion and memory.

Bilateral hippocampal damage, whether from surgical resection, stroke, anoxia, or neurodegenerative disease, produces profound anterograde amnesia with preservation of remote memories and procedural learning. The vulnerability of hippocampal CA1 neurons to hypoxic-ischemic injury makes this region particularly susceptible to damage following cardiac arrest or severe hypotension.

Amygdala

The amygdala is an almond-shaped nuclear complex located directly lateral to the uncus, anterior and superior to the hippocampus, from which it is separated by the anterior end of the temporal horn of the lateral ventricle. The amygdala directs hypothalamic functions related to emotional responses and comprises three major nuclear groups, all extensively interconnected:

Medial Nuclei—Involved in olfactory processing, receiving direct connections from the olfactory tracts.

Central Nucleus—Mediates physiological responses to emotion, receiving connections from the hypothalamus and septal nuclei via the stria terminalis. The central nucleus sends outputs to the hippocampus via both the stria terminalis and ventral amygdalofugal pathways, enabling emotional modulation of memory formation.

Basolateral Nuclear Group—Processes the emotional context of memory and weighs the significance of memories. This largest amygdalar subdivision receives input from the hippocampus, association cortices, basal forebrain (supporting awareness), and thalamus via ventral amygdalofugal pathways. It sends outputs to the hippocampus (to direct memory consolidation), association cortices, ascending reticular activating system (ARAS) and interpeduncular nucleus (affecting awareness and attention), basal forebrain, cingulate gyrus (influencing decision-making and emotional experience), and hypothalamus.

Amygdalar Pathways

Stria Terminalis

This bidirectional fiber bundle serves as an analog of the fornix for the amygdala, connecting it with the septal nuclei, lateral hypothalamus, thalamus (dorsomedial nucleus), caudate-putamen, ventral striatum, and preoptic areas.

Ventral Amygdalofugal Pathway

These fibers pass beneath the lenticular nucleus and spread widely across the basal forebrain, terminating in the septal nuclei, hypothalamus (via the entorhinal cortex), anterior olfactory nucleus, anterior perforated substance (including the substantia innominata), piriform cortex, orbital cortex, anterior cingulate cortex, ventral striatum (nucleus accumbens), and dorsomedial thalamus.

Rapid Emotional Response System

The amygdala participates in a rapid subcortical pathway for emotional responses. Emotionally significant stimuli (such as a threatening sound like a police siren) reach the sensory thalamus and unimodal association areas, which trigger the amygdala. The amygdala then activates the hypothalamus via the central nucleus, initiating arousal and sympathetic nervous system responses before conscious cortical processing is complete. Polymodal association cortex can subsequently modulate or terminate this system after more detailed analysis. This dual-pathway system enables both rapid defensive responses and more nuanced emotional reactions informed by context and memory.

Fornix

The fornix is a prominent C-shaped fiber bundle that connects the hippocampus with the mammillary bodies, anterior thalamic nuclei, and septal nuclei. This bidirectional pathway is essential for memory processing and spatial navigation, carrying hippocampal output to downstream limbic structures and providing reciprocal connections that modulate hippocampal function.

Mammillary Bodies

These paired spherical structures protrude from the ventral hypothalamus at the base of the brain and form a key node in the Papez circuit, which links the hippocampus, fornix, mammillary bodies, anterior thalamic nuclei, cingulate cortex, and back to the hippocampus. Damage to the mammillary bodies, as occurs in Wernicke-Korsakoff syndrome secondary to thiamine deficiency, produces severe memory impairment, particularly affecting the formation of new memories.

Septal Nuclei

Located near the anterior commissure in the medial frontal lobe, the septal nuclei participate in reward processing, reinforcement learning, emotional regulation, and autonomic function. These structures connect extensively with the hippocampus and other limbic regions, contributing to motivation and the experience of pleasure.

Limbic Basal Ganglia

The ventral striatum (including the nucleus accumbens) and ventral pallidum represent limbic components of the basal ganglia that integrate emotional and motivational information with motor control. The nucleus accumbens is a critical node in the brain's reward circuit and plays central roles in addiction, motivation, and reinforcement learning.

Hypothalamus

Although not technically part of the limbic cortex, the hypothalamus is functionally integrated with the limbic system through extensive reciprocal connections. It translates emotional and motivational states into autonomic, endocrine, and behavioral responses. The hypothalamus regulates fundamental survival behaviors including feeding, drinking, thermoregulation, sleep-wake cycles, and reproduction. It controls the autonomic nervous system and, via the pituitary gland, regulates the endocrine system.

Functional Roles of the Limbic System

Emotion Generation and Regulation

The limbic system orchestrates emotional experiences and responses. The amygdala rapidly evaluates the emotional significance of stimuli and triggers appropriate physiological and behavioral responses through its connections with the hypothalamus and brainstem. The cingulate cortex and prefrontal regions modulate these responses, integrating emotional reactions with cognitive appraisal, contextual information, and social norms.

Memory Formation and Consolidation

The hippocampus and surrounding medial temporal structures are indispensable for encoding new declarative memories. The hippocampus binds together distributed cortical representations into coherent memory traces and coordinates their consolidation into long-term storage in neocortex. The entorhinal cortex serves as the primary gateway for cortical information entering and leaving the hippocampus. The Papez circuit links memory formation with emotional processing, explaining why emotionally significant events are often better remembered than neutral experiences.

Motivation and Reward Processing

The ventral striatum, particularly the nucleus accumbens, processes reward signals and mediates motivated behavior. This system evaluates the rewarding properties of stimuli and actions, driving approach behaviors toward beneficial outcomes. The septal nuclei contribute to positive reinforcement and the experience of pleasure. Dysregulation of these circuits contributes to addiction, in which natural reward processing becomes hijacked by drugs or compulsive behaviors.

Autonomic and Endocrine Regulation

The limbic system, particularly through its connections with the hypothalamus, coordinates autonomic and endocrine responses to emotional states and homeostatic challenges. The hypothalamic-pituitary-adrenal (HPA) axis mediates stress responses, releasing cortisol and other stress hormones. Emotional experiences activate the sympathetic nervous system, producing changes in heart rate, blood pressure, respiration, and other visceral functions that prepare the organism for action.

Clinical Disorders of the Limbic System

Mood Disorders

Major depressive disorder and bipolar disorder involve dysregulation of limbic circuits. Structural and functional abnormalities have been documented in the hippocampus, amygdala, anterior cingulate cortex, and prefrontal regions. Reduced hippocampal volume is frequently observed in chronic depression, while amygdalar hyperactivity may contribute to emotional dysregulation and negative biases in emotional processing.

Anxiety Disorders

Post-traumatic stress disorder (PTSD), generalized anxiety disorder, panic disorder, and specific phobias all involve abnormal limbic function. Amygdalar hyperreactivity to threat-related stimuli is a common finding, while reduced prefrontal control over limbic responses may contribute to persistent anxiety and fear. In PTSD, contextual fear conditioning mediated by hippocampal-amygdalar interactions produces intrusive re-experiencing of traumatic memories and exaggerated startle responses.

Memory Disorders

Hippocampal damage produces anterograde amnesia regardless of etiology. Alzheimer's disease characteristically begins with entorhinal cortex and hippocampal degeneration, producing insidious memory decline that progresses to widespread cognitive impairment. Korsakoff syndrome from mammillary body damage produces amnesia with prominent confabulation. Herpes simplex encephalitis has a predilection for medial temporal structures, often producing severe amnesia in survivors. Transient global amnesia, though self-limited, may reflect temporary hippocampal dysfunction.

Alzheimer's Disease: Pathophysiology and Clinical Correlates

Alzheimer's disease represents the most common neurodegenerative disorder and the leading cause of dementia worldwide. Understanding its molecular pathogenesis, staging, and clinical manifestations is essential for neurological practice.

Neuropathological Hallmarks

Alzheimer's disease is characterized by extracellular amyloid plaques composed of aggregated amyloid-beta (Aβ) peptide and intracellular neurofibrillary tangles composed of hyperphosphorylated tau protein. Additional pathological features include amyloid angiopathy (amyloid deposition in cerebral blood vessels), dystrophic neurites, progressive neuronal death, synaptic loss, and deficits in cholinergic and glutamatergic neurotransmission.

The disease follows a predictable anatomical progression described by the Braak staging system. In Transentorhinal Stages (I-II), pathology is limited to the transentorhinal region. In Limbic Stages (III-IV), the disease extends to the hippocampus and adjacent limbic structures, producing clinically evident memory impairment. In Neocortical Stages (V-VI), pathology spreads to association cortices and eventually primary sensory and motor areas. Notably, primary motor and sensory cortices (precentral and postcentral gyri) are relatively spared until late stages, which accounts for the typical clinical presentation of cognitive decline without prominent motor or sensory deficits.

Molecular Pathogenesis

Amyloid Precursor Protein (APP) Processing

APP is a transmembrane protein encoded on chromosome 21, which explains why individuals with Down syndrome (trisomy 21) invariably develop Alzheimer's pathology by middle age. APP can be cleaved by different secretases: α-secretase produces non-amyloidogenic fragments, while sequential cleavage by β-secretase and γ-secretase (a multiprotein complex including presenilin 1 and presenilin 2) generates Aβ peptides, particularly the pathogenic 42-amino acid species (Aβ42).

Excitotoxicity

Glutamate excitotoxicity contributes to neuronal death in Alzheimer's disease. Excessive glutamate receptor activation, particularly of NMDA receptors with high calcium permeability, leads to intracellular calcium overload. When the sodium/potassium gradient fails (as in ischemia or energy depletion), membrane depolarization removes magnesium blockade from NMDA receptors, facilitating massive calcium influx. Additional calcium entry through TRP channels and acid-sensing ion channels (ASIC) further amplifies calcium-mediated calcium release from intracellular stores.

Elevated intracellular calcium activates destructive enzymes, including calpains (proteases), phospholipases, endonucleases, and various kinases, causing cellular destruction. This process generates reactive oxygen species (ROS) and reactive nitrogen species (RNS), particularly peroxynitrite formed when nitric oxide (NO) reacts with superoxide anions. Nitric oxide is synthesized by calcium-dependent neuronal nitric oxide synthase (nNOS), and peroxynitrite promotes extensive tissue damage.

Metabotropic glutamate receptors (mGluRs) also participate in excitotoxicity. Group I mGluRs enhance neuronal excitability by downregulating potassium channels, upregulating non-selective cation channels, inhibiting GABA receptors, and potentiating ionotropic glutamate receptor function. Group II and III mGluRs, located presynaptically, modulate glutamate and GABA release.

Glutamate transporters normally maintain steep glutamate gradients between intracellular and extracellular compartments. EAAT2 (GLT1), expressed on neurons and astrocytes, co-transports three sodium ions and one proton while anti-transporting one potassium ion with each glutamate molecule. During ischemia, dissipation of sodium/potassium gradients impairs or even reverses these transporters, potentially releasing glutamate and exacerbating excitotoxicity. Glutamate sources during pathological conditions include vesicular release, reversed glutamate transporters, necrotic cell death, vesicular release from activated astrocytes and microglia, and furosemide-sensitive release through volume-regulated anion channels (VRAC/VSOAC). Certain neuronal populations are particularly vulnerable, including CA1 hippocampal pyramidal neurons, striatal medium spiny neurons, and spinal cord motor neurons.

Genetics of Alzheimer's Disease

Mutations in APP cause approximately 0.1% of Alzheimer's cases. Missense mutations in presenilin 1 (PSEN1) and presenilin 2 (PSEN2) genes cause early-onset autosomal dominant Alzheimer's disease by altering γ-secretase activity to favor production of the more aggregation-prone Aβ42 species. Apolipoprotein E (APOE) polymorphisms represent the strongest genetic risk factor for late-onset sporadic Alzheimer's disease. The APOE ε4 allele increases aggregation and decreases clearance of Aβ42, substantially elevating disease risk, while the ε2 allele is protective.

Therapeutic Strategies

Current and investigational therapeutic approaches target various aspects of Alzheimer's pathophysiology:

- Inhibiting β-secretase or γ-secretase to reduce Aβ production
- Enhancing Aβ clearance using anti-Aβ antibodies (passive immunotherapy) or Aβ vaccines (active immunotherapy)
- Preventing Aβ aggregation using small molecule inhibitors
- Inhibiting neuroinflammatory processes in the brain
- Interfering with downstream toxic responses including excitotoxicity, oxidative stress, and apoptosis

The Insula: Interoception, Emotion, and Self-Awareness

The insula (Island of Reil) is a distinct cortical region hidden within the lateral (Sylvian) fissure, concealed by the overlying frontal, parietal, and temporal opercula. Despite its hidden location, the insula performs critical functions in interoception (perception of internal bodily states), emotional processing, autonomic regulation, pain perception, and self-awareness, making it essential for integrating bodily signals with emotional and cognitive states.

Anatomical Organization

Anterior Insula

The anterior insula integrates emotional and bodily states into higher-order cognitive processing. It maintains extensive connections with the prefrontal cortex, enabling contributions to emotional regulation, decision-making, and cognitive control. This region processes interoceptive signals about internal body states (hunger, thirst, pain, arousal) and generates conscious awareness of these sensations. The anterior insula is also central to empathy and social cognition, allowing us to simulate others' emotional experiences within our own neural and bodily systems.

Posterior Insula

The posterior insula processes primary sensory information from the body, including somatosensory inputs (pain, temperature, touch) and visceral sensations from internal organs. This region integrates respiratory and cardiovascular signals, contributing to the perception and regulation of autonomic states. The posterior insula provides the raw sensory substrate that the anterior insula then integrates into conscious awareness and emotional experience.

Functional Roles of the Insula

Interoception and Bodily Awareness

The insula serves as the primary cortical center for interoception—the sense of the physiological condition of the body. It processes signals from visceral organs, muscles, skin, and the vestibular system, generating conscious awareness of internal states, including hunger, thirst, pain, temperature, cardiac rhythm, respiratory effort, and even the subjective experience of being immersed in a task ("flow"). This continuous monitoring of bodily states is essential for maintaining homeostasis and responding adaptively to the body's needs.

Emotional Processing and Regulation

The anterior insula integrates visceral signals with emotional states, generating the subjective feeling component of emotions. It is particularly active during experiences of disgust, fear, anger, and anxiety. The insula helps generate emotion-related bodily sensations—the racing heart, sweating palms, or visceral "gut feelings" that accompany emotional experiences. This integration of bodily and emotional signals allows emotions to be experienced as embodied phenomena rather than purely cognitive events.

Social Cognition and Empathy

The insula enables empathy by allowing us to simulate others' emotional and bodily states within our own neural systems. When observing another person in pain or distress, the insula activates in patterns similar to experiencing those states directly. This neural resonance provides the foundation for empathic understanding and appropriate social responses. The insula contributes to self-awareness and self-reflection by integrating bodily sensations and emotional experiences into our sense of self.

Autonomic Regulation

Through extensive connections with hypothalamic and brainstem autonomic centers, the insula influences sympathetic and parasympathetic nervous system activity. It integrates visceral sensory information with emotional states and cognitive demands to modulate heart rate, blood pressure, respiration, and gastrointestinal function. This bidirectional communication allows emotional and cognitive states to influence autonomic function while autonomic signals shape emotional experience.

Decision-Making and Risk Processing

The anterior insula participates in decision-making, particularly under conditions of uncertainty, risk, or potential negative outcomes. It processes the affective value of potential outcomes and becomes especially active when evaluating risky choices or potential losses. This region helps integrate emotional signals ("gut feelings") into rational decision-making processes, enabling more adaptive choices that consider both logical analysis and emotional/bodily responses.

Clinical Disorders Involving the Insula

Emotional and Psychiatric Disorders

Insular dysfunction contributes to numerous psychiatric conditions. Anxiety disorders, including generalized anxiety disorder, panic disorder, and PTSD, involve anterior insular hyperactivity and heightened sensitivity to interoceptive signals. Depression is associated with altered insular function affecting emotional processing and reactivity. Borderline personality disorder involves insular abnormalities related to emotional awareness and regulation.

Pain Disorders

The insula's central role in pain processing makes it relevant to chronic pain conditions. Dysregulation of insular activity contributes to fibromyalgia, complex regional pain syndrome, and other chronic pain states. Abnormal insular processing may produce allodynia (pain from normally innocuous stimuli) and hyperalgesia (increased sensitivity to painful stimuli).

Addiction

The insula plays a crucial role in drug craving and addiction. Remarkably, damage to the insula can eliminate cigarette cravings in smokers, suggesting that this region is necessary for maintaining addictive behavior. The insula may process the interoceptive signals associated with drug withdrawal and craving, perpetuating the addiction cycle.

Autism Spectrum Disorder and Schizophrenia

Insular dysfunction may contribute to social cognitive deficits in autism spectrum disorder, affecting empathy and emotional understanding. In schizophrenia, altered insular activity has been associated with social dysfunction, emotional dysregulation, and auditory hallucinations.

Autonomic Dysfunction

The insula's role in autonomic regulation makes it relevant to conditions involving autonomic dysregulation. Irritable bowel syndrome involves misprocessing of gut sensations, while neurocardiogenic syncope may reflect abnormal insular regulation of cardiovascular responses.

Cortical Communications: White Matter Pathways

The functional integration of diverse cortical regions depends on an elaborate system of white matter pathways that connect different cortical areas with each other and with subcortical structures. Understanding these connections is essential for predicting the consequences of focal brain lesions.

Intracortical Communications

Intracortical connections typically arise from layer III neurons and terminate in the supragranular layers (I, II, and III) of target cortical regions. These connections can be subdivided into several categories:

Commissural Fibers

Commissural fibers cross between hemispheres through the corpus callosum (connecting most cortical areas) and the anterior commissure (connecting anterior temporal and olfactory regions). These connections enable interhemispheric communication and coordinate processing between homologous regions of the two hemispheres.

Association Fibers

Association fibers connect different cortical regions within the same hemisphere and include several major fasciculi:

- *Superior Longitudinal Fasciculus*—connects frontal and parietal lobes
- *Arcuate Fasciculus*—connects Broca's and Wernicke's areas, essential for language
- *Inferior Fronto-occipital Fasciculus*—links frontal and occipital regions
- *Uncinate Fasciculus*—connects frontal and anterior temporal regions
- *Inferior Longitudinal Fasciculus*—runs along the temporal lobe
- *Cingulum*—courses within the cingulate gyrus, linking limbic structures
- *Short Association Fibers*—connect adjacent gyri within a lobe

Subcortical Communications

The centrum semiovale represents the white matter exiting from cortical gray matter, which eventually becomes the corona radiata as fibers converge toward the internal capsule. Major subcortical projection systems include:

Thalamocortical and Corticothalamic Fibers—Corticothalamic projections originate in layer VI; thalamocortical afferents terminate primarily in layer IV, with the density of these projections visible as Baillarger's lines in sensory cortices.

Corticostriatal Fibers—Arise from layer V and project to the caudate nucleus and putamen, forming critical loops for motor control and habit learning.

Motor System Projections—Corticospinal and corticobulbar fibers originate in layer V, particularly from the primary motor cortex, premotor areas, and supplementary motor area.

Diffuse Projection Systems—Ascending modulatory systems from the brainstem (cholinergic, noradrenergic, serotonergic, dopaminergic) terminate diffusely across all cortical layers, regulating arousal, attention, and mood.

Vascular Supply and Stroke Syndromes

Middle Cerebral Artery Territory

The middle cerebral artery (MCA) supplies the lateral convexity of the cerebral hemispheres, including critical functional areas (Figs. 7.3 and 7.4). MCA infarction produces characteristic clinical syndromes depending on the hemisphere affected:

Broca's Area (left) or *motor prosody (right)*—expressive language impairment or loss of emotional inflection

Frontal Eye Fields—ipsilateral gaze deviation (eyes look toward the lesion)

Precentral Gyrus—contralateral hemiparesis affecting face and upper extremity more than leg

Postcentral Gyrus—contralateral hemisensory loss

Wernicke's Area (left) or *receptive prosody (right)*—language comprehension deficit or inability to comprehend emotional tone

Primary Auditory Cortex—no complete hearing loss due to bilateral representation, but sound localization deficits may occur

Parietal Lobe—neglect syndromes (especially with right hemisphere lesions)

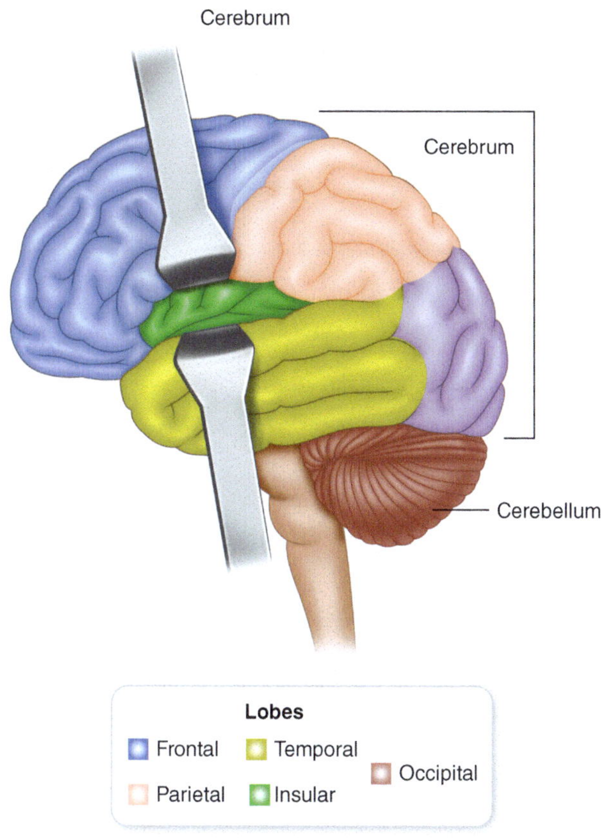

Fig. 7.3 Lateral view of the cerebrum with color-coded lobes, illustrating the five principal lobes of the cerebral hemisphere: frontal (blue), parietal (pink), temporal (yellow), insular (green), and occipital (purple). The cerebellum is visible inferoposteriorly

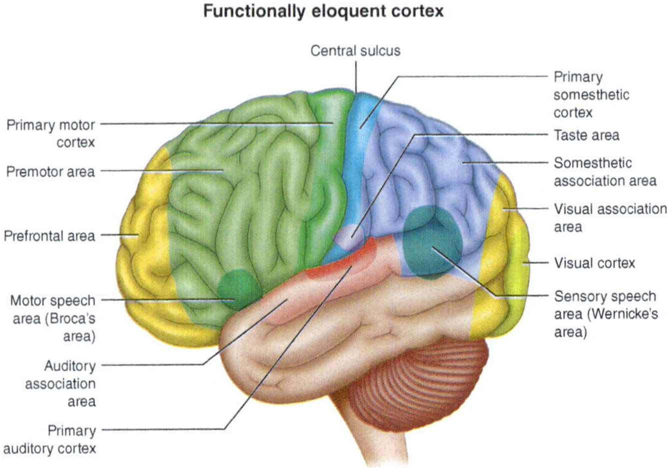

Fig. 7.4 Lateral view of the left cerebral hemisphere illustrating the functionally eloquent cortical areas, including the primary motor cortex and premotor area (anterior to the central sulcus), primary somesthetic cortex and somesthetic association area (posterior to the central sulcus), primary auditory cortex and auditory association area (superior temporal gyrus), primary visual cortex and visual association area (occipital lobe), motor speech area (Broca's area, inferior frontal gyrus), sensory speech area (Wernicke's area, posterior superior temporal gyrus), taste area, and prefrontal area

Venous Drainage

Cortical veins drain into dural venous sinuses through superficial and deep systems:

Superficial Veins

The superior anastomotic vein of Trolard, inferior anastomotic vein of Labbé, and superficial middle cerebral vein drain into the superior sagittal sinus and transverse sinus.

Deep Veins

The basal vein of Rosenthal, internal cerebral veins, and inferior sagittal sinus converge to form the great cerebral vein of Galen.

Clinical Syndromes: Aphasias and Disconnection Syndromes

Classification of Aphasias

Aphasias can be systematically classified based on fluency, comprehension, and repetition abilities. Understanding these patterns enables anatomical localization of lesions:

Transcortical Sensory Aphasia—lesion: cortical connections to Wernicke's area; comprehension: impaired; fluency: fluent; repetition: preserved

Wernicke's Aphasia—lesion: Wernicke's area; comprehension: impaired; fluency: fluent; repetition: impaired

Conduction Aphasia—lesion: arcuate fasciculus; comprehension: preserved; fluency: fluent; repetition: severely impaired

Broca's Aphasia—lesion: Broca's area; comprehension: preserved; fluency: non-fluent; repetition: impaired

Transcortical Motor Aphasia—lesion: cortical connections to Broca's area; comprehension: preserved; fluency: non-fluent; repetition: preserved

Global Aphasia—lesion: Broca's and Wernicke's areas; comprehension: impaired; fluency: non-fluent; repetition: impaired

Disconnection Syndromes

Disconnection syndromes result from damage to white matter pathways that link functional cortical regions, producing deficits despite intact primary cortical areas:

Corpus Callosotomy

Surgical division of the corpus callosum produces visual disconnection. Objects presented in the left visual field can be drawn with the left hand (controlled by the right hemisphere) but cannot be verbally identified because language centers in the left hemisphere lack access to right hemisphere visual information. Objects in the right visual field can be identified verbally because visual information reaches the left hemisphere directly.

Alexia Without Agraphia
Combined damage to the left visual cortex and the posterior corpus callosum (splenium) disconnects right hemisphere visual information from left hemisphere language areas, producing an inability to read despite preserved writing ability.

Geschwind's Disconnection Syndromes
Norman Geschwind described numerous disconnection syndromes resulting from specific white matter lesions:

Apraxia—disconnection of parietal association cortex from frontal association cortex
Tactile Aphasia—disconnection of somatosensory cortex from Wernicke's area
Tactile Agnosia—disconnection of somatosensory cortex from parietal association cortex
Pure Word Deafness—disconnection of auditory cortex from Wernicke's area
Verbal Learning Impairment—disconnection of auditory cortex from limbic system
Pain Asymbolia—disconnection of somatosensory cortex from limbic system
Pure Alexia—disconnection of visual cortex from parietal association areas
Visual Agnosia—disconnection of visual cortex from parietal association areas

Neurodegenerative Patterns

Frontotemporal Dementia (Pick's Disease)
This tauopathy selectively affects frontal and temporal lobes while sparing parietal and occipital regions. Clinical manifestations include progressive behavioral changes, personality alterations, and language dysfunction.

Alzheimer's Disease
Characteristically involves association cortices before primary sensory and motor areas. The brain often shows generalized atrophy with relatively preserved precentral and postcentral gyri, reflecting the disease's predilection for association cortex and limbic structures.

Amyotrophic Lateral Sclerosis
Selective degeneration of upper motor neurons produces marked atrophy of the precentral gyrus while the postcentral gyrus remains relatively preserved, creating a distinctive imaging appearance.

Conclusion

The cerebral cortex represents the anatomical foundation for uniquely human cognitive capabilities, orchestrating the perception, integration, and generation of the vast repertoire of behaviors that define human experience. Its systematic organization into functionally specialized regions, interconnected through elaborate white matter pathways and integrated with subcortical structures, enables the remarkable computational power of the human brain.

Understanding cortical neuroanatomy provides the essential framework for clinical practice. The principles of cortical localization—refined since the pioneering observations of Broca, Wernicke, and Brodmann—remain fundamental to neurological diagnosis. Recognizing patterns of cortical dysfunction allows clinicians to localize lesions, predict deficits, and understand the anatomical basis of neurological and psychiatric disease.

The cortex's remarkable plasticity offers hope for recovery after injury and continues to inspire novel therapeutic approaches for neurological disease. As our understanding of cortical organization and function deepens through advanced neuroimaging, molecular biology, and systems neuroscience, the classical anatomical knowledge presented in this chapter provides the enduring foundation upon which modern neuroscience and clinical neurology are built.

Mastery of cortical neuroanatomy equips medical students and residents with the knowledge necessary to understand normal brain function, recognize patterns of disease, and provide compassionate, informed care to patients with neurological disorders. This anatomical foundation, integrated with physiological understanding and clinical experience, forms the cornerstone of competent neurological practice.

The Ventricular System and Hydrocephalus

8

Introduction

The cerebral ventricles constitute a sophisticated system of interconnected, fluid-filled cavities located within the brain parenchyma (Fig. 8.1). These structures form the ventricular system, which serves critical functions in producing, circulating, and removing cerebrospinal fluid (CSF). CSF provides mechanical protection to neural tissue, delivers essential nutrients to brain structures, and facilitates waste removal from the central nervous system. The ventricles are strategically positioned within the cerebral hemispheres, brainstem, and spinal cord. Their walls are lined with specialized ependymal cells, which play crucial roles in both CSF production and circulation.

V. Yanamadala, *Essential Neuroanatomy*,
https://doi.org/10.1007/978-3-032-26877-8_8

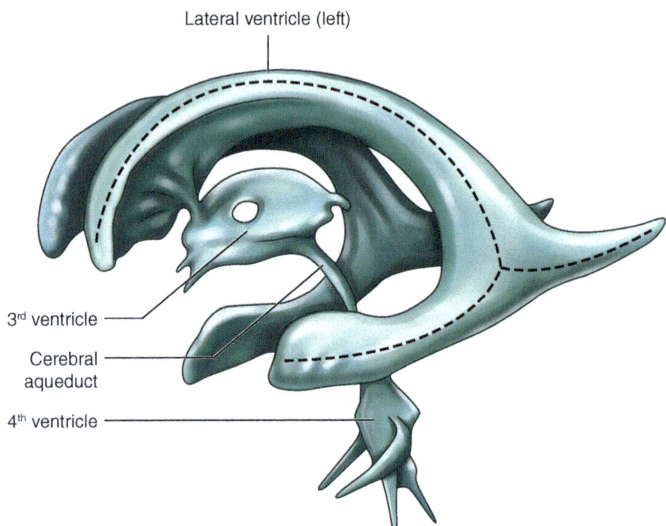

Fig. 8.1 Three-dimensional rendering of the ventricular system viewed from the left lateral perspective, demonstrating the spatial relationships of the lateral ventricle (left), third ventricle, cerebral aqueduct, and fourth ventricle

Anatomical Components of the Ventricular System

The ventricular system consists of five interconnected structures that form a continuous pathway for CSF circulation. Understanding each component's anatomy is essential for comprehending normal CSF dynamics and recognizing pathological conditions.

Lateral Ventricles

The lateral ventricles represent the largest components of the ventricular system, with one present in each cerebral hemisphere. These paired structures exhibit a characteristic C-shaped configuration that mirrors the developmental curvature of the cerebral hemispheres.

Anatomical Organization Each lateral ventricle consists of a central body and three extensions termed horns. The anterior horn (frontal horn) projects into the frontal lobe, extending anteriorly and laterally. The posterior horn (occipital horn) extends posteriorly into the occipital lobe, though it is often smaller and more variable in size. The inferior horn (temporal horn) curves inferolaterally into the temporal lobe, following the arc of the hippocampus.

Choroid Plexus The lateral ventricles contain prominent choroid plexus, a specialized structure composed of highly vascularized connective tissue covered by ependymal cells. This structure produces the majority of CSF in the brain. The choroid plexus is most abundant in the body and inferior horn of the lateral ventricles, where it forms an elongated, frond-like structure.

Interventricular Foramen Also known as the foramen of Monro, this narrow passageway connects each lateral ventricle to the third ventricle. Bilateral interventricular foramina exist, positioned at the anterior-superior aspect of the third ventricle. These openings are clinically significant as their obstruction can lead to unilateral or bilateral ventricular enlargement.

Third Ventricle

The third ventricle is a narrow, slit-like midline cavity located within the diencephalon. It occupies the space between the two thalami and lies inferior to the corpus callosum. This ventricle has a roughly triangular shape when viewed sagittally, with its long axis oriented in the anteroposterior direction. The walls of the third ventricle are formed medially by the thalami, with the hypothalamus forming its floor. A small portion of choroid plexus exists in the roof of the third ventricle, though it is less prominent than in the lateral ventricles. The third ventricle communicates anteriorly with the lateral ventricles through the interventricular foramina and posteriorly with the fourth ventricle via the cerebral aqueduct.

Cerebral Aqueduct (Aqueduct of Sylvius)

The cerebral aqueduct, also designated the aqueduct of Sylvius, is a narrow conduit coursing through the midbrain. This tubular structure, approximately 2–3 centimeters in length in adults, passes through the tectum (the dorsal midbrain) and connects the third ventricle superiorly to the fourth ventricle inferiorly. Despite its small caliber, the cerebral aqueduct is a critical passage for CSF flow. Aqueductal stenosis, whether congenital or acquired, represents the most common site of obstruction in noncommunicating hydrocephalus, resulting in dilation of the upstream lateral and third ventricles.

Fourth Ventricle

The fourth ventricle occupies a position in the posterior fossa, bounded anteriorly by the pons and medulla oblongata and posteriorly by the cerebellum. This ventricle exhibits a characteristic diamond or tent-shaped appearance, with its apex directed superiorly toward the cerebral aqueduct and its base oriented inferiorly. The fourth ventricle represents a critical juncture in CSF circulation as it provides the principal exit route for CSF from the ventricular system into the subarachnoid space. Choroid plexus is present in the roof of the fourth ventricle, particularly near the foramen of Magendie. Three apertures allow CSF egress from the fourth ventricle: the midline foramen of Magendie (median aperture) and the paired lateral foramina of Luschka (lateral apertures). These openings permit CSF to flow into the subarachnoid space surrounding the brain and spinal cord.

Central Canal of the Spinal Cord

The central canal represents the caudal continuation of the ventricular system, extending throughout the length of the spinal cord from the fourth ventricle to the conus medullaris. This narrow, ependymal-lined channel allows CSF to circulate within the spinal cord, contributing to spinal cord buoyancy, nutrient delivery, and waste removal. In adults, portions of the central canal may become obliterated, though it typically remains patent in the cervical and upper thoracic regions.

Cerebrospinal Fluid Dynamics

CSF Production Cerebrospinal fluid is primarily produced by the choroid plexus within the lateral ventricles, with smaller contributions from the choroid plexus in the third and fourth ventricles. The choroid plexus produces approximately 500 milliliters of CSF daily in adults, though only about 150 milliliters are present in the ventricular system and subarachnoid space at any given time, necessitating complete CSF turnover multiple times per day.

Circulation Pathway CSF flows in a precisely orchestrated sequence depicted in Fig. 8.2. From the lateral ventricles, CSF passes through the interventricular foramina (foramina of Monro) into the third ventricle. The fluid then traverses the cerebral aqueduct (aqueduct of Sylvius) to reach the fourth ventricle. From the fourth ventricle, CSF exits the ventricular system through the foramen of Magendie and foramina of Luschka, entering the subarachnoid space. Within the subarachnoid space, CSF circulates around the brain and spinal cord, bathing the external surfaces of the central nervous system. Finally, CSF is reabsorbed into the venous circulation through arachnoid villi (also called arachnoid granulations), specialized structures that protrude into the dural venous sinuses, particularly the superior sagittal sinus.

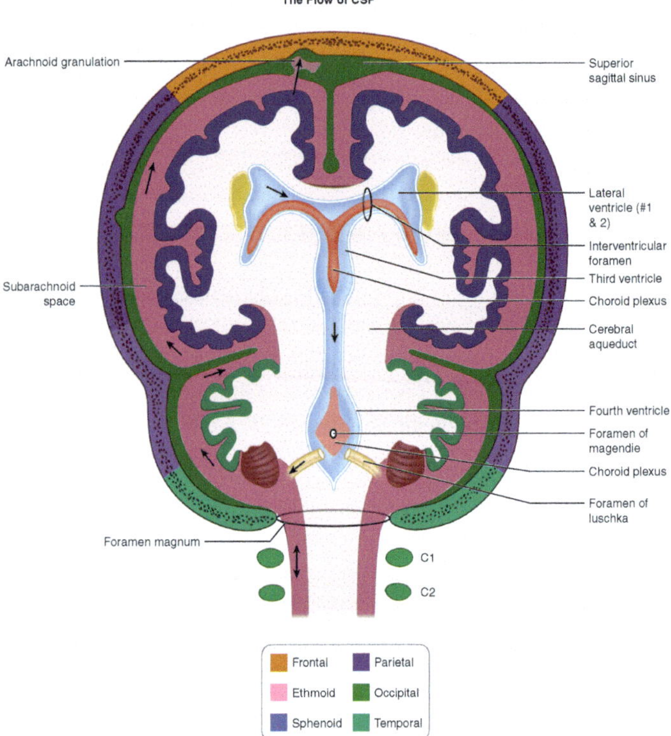

Fig. 8.2 Coronal section of the brain and upper cervical spinal cord illustrating the circulation of cerebrospinal fluid (CSF), from its production at the choroid plexus through the ventricular system (lateral, third, and fourth ventricles), foramina of Luschka and Magendie, subarachnoid space, and reabsorption at the arachnoid granulations into the superior sagittal sinus. A color-coded key identifies the overlying cranial bones

Hydrocephalus

Hydrocephalus, derived from Greek words meaning water (hydro) and head (cephalus), is a neurological condition characterized by abnormal accumulation of cerebrospinal fluid within the ventricular system. This accumulation typically leads to ventricular enlargement and increased intracranial pressure, potentially causing compression of brain tissue and neurological dysfunction. Hydrocephalus may occur at any age and arises from various etiologies. Understanding its classification, pathophysiology, and clinical manifestations is essential for appropriate diagnosis and management.

Classification of Hydrocephalus

Communicating Hydrocephalus

Communicating hydrocephalus occurs when CSF can flow freely through the ventricular system but encounters impaired reabsorption into the venous circulation. In this form, the pathways connecting all ventricles remain patent, including the foramina of Monro, cerebral aqueduct, and fourth ventricular outlets. The obstruction to CSF flow occurs distal to these structures, typically at the level of the arachnoid villi in the subarachnoid space. Common etiologies include meningitis, subarachnoid hemorrhage, meningeal carcinomatosis, and elevated venous sinus pressure. These conditions can damage or obstruct the arachnoid villi, preventing adequate CSF reabsorption despite normal production rates.

Non-communicating (Obstructive) Hydrocephalus

Non-communicating hydrocephalus, also termed obstructive hydrocephalus, results from blockage within the ventricular system itself, preventing CSF from reaching the subarachnoid space for normal reabsorption. The most common site of obstruction is the cerebral aqueduct (aqueduct of Sylvius), where stenosis leads to isolated dilation of the lateral and third ventricles while the fourth ventricle remains normal in size. Obstruction of the interventricular foramina (foramina of Monro) can cause unilateral or bilateral lateral ventricular enlargement with normal third and fourth ventricles.

Multiple pathological processes can cause non-communicating hydrocephalus. Congenital aqueductal stenosis represents an important cause in pediatric patients. Brain tumors, particularly those in the posterior fossa or pineal region, can compress the aqueduct or fourth ventricular outlets. Cysts, including colloid cysts of the third ventricle, may obstruct the foramina of Monro. Infections such as meningitis or tuberculosis can cause inflammatory adhesions that obstruct CSF pathways. Traumatic brain injury may result in hemorrhage or scarring that impedes CSF flow.

Normal Pressure Hydrocephalus

Normal pressure hydrocephalus (NPH) represents a unique form of communicating hydrocephalus predominantly affecting older adults. This condition is characterized by gradual ventricular enlargement occurring without sustained elevation of intracranial pressure, hence the designation as normal pressure. NPH classically presents with the Hakim-Adams triad: gait disturbance (typically a magnetic, shuffling gait with difficulty initiating walking), urinary incontinence (ranging from urgency to frank incontinence), and cognitive impairment (featuring memory problems and executive dysfunction). The underlying pathophysiology involves impaired CSF absorption, though the mechanism allowing ventricular enlargement without sustained pressure elevation remains incompletely understood. NPH may be idiopathic or secondary to previous brain injury, subarachnoid hemorrhage, or meningitis.

Congenital Hydrocephalus

Congenital hydrocephalus is present at birth and stems from genetic mutations, intrauterine infections, or developmental brain malformations. Common causes include aqueductal stenosis, which may occur as an isolated finding or as part of genetic syndromes. Chiari malformation type II, frequently associated with myelomeningocele, often causes fourth ventricular obstruction. Dandy-Walker malformation, characterized by partial or complete agenesis of the cerebellar vermis and cystic dilation of the fourth ventricle, commonly results in hydrocephalus. Neural tube defects, particularly myelomeningocele (spina bifida), are frequently accompanied by hydrocephalus requiring shunt placement.

Acquired Hydrocephalus

Acquired hydrocephalus develops after birth in response to brain injury, infection, hemorrhage, or mass lesions. Traumatic brain injury, particularly when accompanied by intraventricular or subarachnoid hemorrhage, may damage CSF pathways or arachnoid villi. Central nervous system infections, including bacterial meningitis and viral encephalitis, can cause inflammatory adhesions obstructing CSF flow. Brain tumors, especially those located in the posterior fossa, pineal region, or third ventricular area, frequently obstruct CSF pathways. Subarachnoid hemorrhage, whether traumatic or aneurysmal, may impair CSF reabsorption at the arachnoid villi through blood product deposition.

Pathophysiology

The ventricular system maintains a delicate balance between CSF production by the choroid plexus and reabsorption through the arachnoid villi. Disruption of this equilibrium leads to hydrocephalus through three principal mechanisms. First, obstruction anywhere along the CSF pathway prevents normal flow, causing accumulation upstream of the blockage. Second, impaired absorption at the arachnoid villi, despite patent CSF pathways, results in ventricular enlargement throughout the system. Third, excessive CSF production, though rare, may overwhelm normal reabsorptive capacity. This typically occurs with choroid plexus tumors (choroid plexus papillomas) that produce CSF at abnormally high rates. The resulting fluid accumulation increases intracranial pressure, compressing and potentially damaging adjacent brain tissue, disrupting normal neurological function.

Clinical Manifestations

The clinical presentation of hydrocephalus varies considerably based on patient age, rate of fluid accumulation, and severity of ventricular enlargement.

Infants and Young Children

In infants, before cranial suture fusion, the skull can expand to accommodate increased intracranial volume. This results in progressive head enlargement (macrocephaly) with accelerated head circumference growth crossing percentiles. The anterior fontanelle becomes tense and bulging. Other manifestations include:

- Prominent scalp veins due to increased venous pressure
- Sunsetting sign (downward deviation of eyes with visible sclera above the iris)
- Irritability and poor feeding
- Vomiting
- Seizures in severe cases
- Developmental delays or regression

Adults and Older Children

In patients with fused cranial sutures, the skull cannot expand, leading to more acute symptoms of increased intracranial pressure:

- Headache, typically worse upon awakening and with Valsalva maneuvers
- Nausea and vomiting, particularly in the morning
- Papilledema (optic disc swelling) visible on fundoscopic examination
- Visual disturbances including blurred vision or diplopia
- Cognitive decline affecting memory, attention, and executive function
- Gait abnormalities ranging from ataxia to apraxia
- Personality changes or behavioral disturbances

Normal Pressure Hydrocephalus Presentation

NPH exhibits a characteristic triad that develops gradually:

- Gait disturbance: Magnetic or shuffling gait with difficulty initiating steps, turning, and maintaining balance
- Urinary symptoms: Urinary urgency progressing to incontinence

- Cognitive impairment: Subcortical dementia pattern with slowed processing, executive dysfunction, and memory retrieval deficits

Diagnosis

Diagnosis of hydrocephalus requires integration of clinical evaluation with neuroimaging studies.

Physical Examination In infants, serial head circumference measurements plotted on growth charts detect abnormal enlargement. Palpation of the fontanelles assesses tension. Fundoscopic examination identifies papilledema in patients with increased intracranial pressure. Neurological examination evaluates cranial nerve function, motor and sensory systems, gait, and cognitive status.

Neuroimaging Computed tomography (CT) and magnetic resonance imaging (MRI) visualize ventricular size and morphology, identify the level of obstruction in non-communicating hydrocephalus, and detect underlying pathology such as tumors, cysts, or malformations. CT provides rapid assessment, making it useful in acute settings. MRI offers superior anatomical detail and multiplanar imaging capabilities. Specific imaging findings help distinguish hydrocephalus from other causes of ventricular enlargement, such as cerebral atrophy.

Additional Studies In selected cases, radionuclide cisternography assesses CSF flow dynamics. For NPH, large-volume lumbar puncture (removal of 30–50 mL CSF) serves both diagnostic and prognostic purposes; improvement in gait following drainage predicts favorable response to shunt surgery. Neuropsychological testing quantifies cognitive deficits and documents improvement following treatment.

Treatment

The primary goal of hydrocephalus treatment is reducing intracranial pressure, restoring normal CSF dynamics, and preventing or minimizing neurological damage.

Surgical Interventions

Ventriculoperitoneal Shunt The most common treatment modality involves implanting a shunt system that diverts CSF from the lateral ventricles to the peritoneal cavity, where it is absorbed. The shunt consists of a ventricular catheter, a valve mechanism to regulate flow and prevent overdrainage, and distal tubing terminating in the peritoneum. Alternative sites for CSF drainage include the right atrium (ventriculoatrial shunt) or pleural space (ventriculopleural shunt). Shunt systems typically function reliably but require lifelong monitoring for potential complications including obstruction, infection, and mechanical failure necessitating revision surgery.

Endoscopic Third Ventriculostomy For selected cases of obstructive hydrocephalus, particularly those with aqueductal stenosis, endoscopic third ventriculostomy (ETV) offers an alternative approach. This minimally invasive procedure creates a fenestration in the floor of the third ventricle, allowing CSF to bypass the obstruction and flow directly to the basal cisterns for reabsorption. ETV avoids permanent foreign body implantation and associated complications. Success rates are highest in patients with obstruction at or below the level of the aqueduct and in older children and adults.

Treatment of Underlying Pathology When hydrocephalus results from an identifiable mass lesion such as a tumor or cyst, surgical removal or reduction of the lesion may alleviate the obstruction and resolve the hydrocephalus, potentially eliminating the need for permanent CSF diversion.

Prognosis and Long-Term Management

With appropriate treatment, many patients with hydrocephalus achieve favorable outcomes. Early diagnosis and intervention are crucial for preventing irreversible neurological damage. Patients with shunt-treated hydrocephalus require lifelong monitoring for signs of shunt malfunction or infection. Shunt revisions are commonly needed, particularly during childhood growth periods. NPH patients who respond to shunt placement may experience significant improvement in gait, cognition, and continence, though response is often incomplete. Overall prognosis depends on etiology, age at onset, duration of symptoms before treatment, and presence of associated neurological conditions.

Conclusion

Understanding the anatomy and physiology of the ventricular system is fundamental to neurology and neurosurgery. The intricate architecture of the lateral ventricles, third ventricle, cerebral aqueduct, fourth ventricle, and central canal, along with their role in CSF production, circulation, and reabsorption, underlies numerous neurological conditions. Hydrocephalus, in its various forms, represents an important clinical manifestation of disrupted CSF dynamics. Recognition of hydrocephalus types, understanding their pathophysiology, and familiarity with diagnostic and therapeutic approaches are essential skills for medical professionals caring for patients with neurological disorders. Continued advances in neuroimaging, neurosurgical techniques, and shunt technology promise improved outcomes for patients affected by these conditions.

9 Blood Supply of the Central Nervous System

Introduction

The blood supply of the brain constitutes a highly organized and intricate vascular network designed to deliver oxygen and nutrients while efficiently removing metabolic waste products from the central nervous system. Despite comprising only 2% of body weight, the brain consumes approximately 20% of the body's oxygen and glucose at rest, underscoring its exceptional metabolic demands and vulnerability to vascular compromise. This chapter examines the anatomical organization, physiological principles, and clinical significance of the central nervous system's blood supply.

The cerebral circulation is primarily served by two major arterial sources: the internal carotid arteries and the vertebral arteries. These vessels give rise to numerous branching arteries that supply distinct regions of the brain. A unique feature of cerebral vasculature is the Circle of Willis (depicted in Fig. 9.1), an anastomotic ring at the base of the brain that provides collateral circulation and helps maintain cerebral perfusion even when one of the major arteries becomes obstructed.

V. Yanamadala, *Essential Neuroanatomy*,
https://doi.org/10.1007/978-3-032-26877-8_9

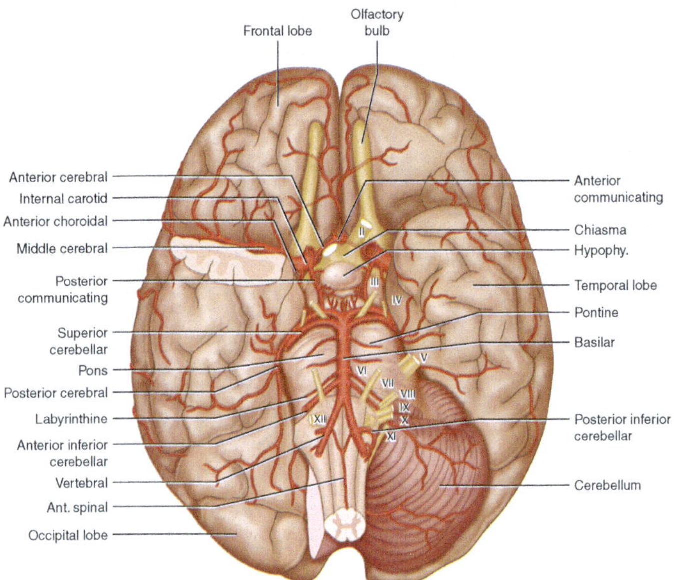

Fig. 9.1 Inferior surface of the brain showing the arterial supply from the circle of Willis and its branches, including the internal carotid, anterior and middle cerebral, anterior and posterior communicating, posterior cerebral, superior cerebellar, basilar, vertebral, and anterior and posterior inferior cerebellar arteries, with cranial nerve roots (II–XII) visible at the brainstem surface

Major Arterial Systems Supplying the Brain

Internal Carotid Arteries

The internal carotid arteries (ICA) arise from the common carotid arteries, which originate from the aortic arch on the left side and the brachiocephalic trunk on the right side. At approximately the level of the C4 vertebra, the common carotid arteries bifurcate into the external and internal carotid arteries. The external carotid artery supplies structures of the face and neck, while the internal carotid artery is dedicated to cerebral perfusion.

After arising from the bifurcation, the internal carotid arteries ascend through the neck and enter the cranial cavity via the carotid canals in the petrous portion of the temporal bone. Within the cavernous sinus, the ICA follows a characteristic S-shaped course (the carotid siphon) before piercing the dura mater to enter the subarachnoid space. This tortuous path may provide some protection against sudden changes in blood pressure.

Major Branches of the Internal Carotid Artery

Ophthalmic Artery This is typically the first major intracranial branch of the ICA, arising as the artery exits the cavernous sinus. It enters the orbit through the optic canal alongside the optic nerve and supplies the eye, extraocular muscles, lacrimal gland, and portions of the nose and forehead. The ophthalmic artery's central retinal artery branch is of particular clinical importance, as occlusion leads to sudden, painless vision loss.

Posterior Communicating Artery This vessel connects the internal carotid artery with the posterior cerebral artery (PCA), forming a crucial component of the Circle of Willis. It provides collateral pathways between the anterior (carotid) and posterior (vertebrobasilar) circulations. The posterior communicating artery gives rise to small perforating branches that supply the thalamus, hypothalamus, and subthalamic region.

Anterior Choroidal Artery This small but clinically significant vessel arises from the ICA just before its terminal bifurcation. It supplies the choroid plexus of the lateral ventricle, portions of the hippocampus, globus pallidus, posterior limb of the internal capsule, and parts of the optic tract. Occlusion can cause contralateral hemiplegia, hemisensory loss, and homonymous hemianopsia—a clinical triad characteristic of anterior choroidal artery syndrome.

Middle Cerebral Artery The middle cerebral artery (MCA) is the largest and most direct continuation of the internal carotid artery. It supplies the lateral aspects of the cerebral hemispheres, including the frontal, parietal, and temporal lobes. The MCA territory encompasses the primary motor and sensory cortices controlling the face, upper extremities, and trunk, as well as critical language areas (Broca's area in the inferior frontal gyrus and Wernicke's area in the superior temporal gyrus) in the dominant hemisphere. The MCA initially courses laterally through the Sylvian fissure, giving off deep penetrating branches (lenticulostriate arteries) that supply the basal ganglia and internal capsule, before dividing into superior and inferior divisions that supply the cortical surface.

Anterior Cerebral Artery The anterior cerebral artery (ACA) is the smaller terminal branch of the internal carotid artery. It supplies the medial aspects of the cerebral hemispheres, including the medial portions of the frontal and parietal lobes. The ACA territory includes the paracentral lobule, which contains the motor and sensory cortices for the lower extremities. The ACA courses medially and anteriorly above the optic chiasm, where it is connected to its contralateral counterpart by the anterior communicating artery. It then curves around the genu of the corpus callosum, giving off the medial lenticulostriate artery (recurrent artery of Heubner), which supplies the head of the caudate nucleus, anterior limb of the internal capsule, and parts of the putamen.

Vertebrobasilar System

The vertebral arteries arise from the subclavian arteries and represent the second major source of cerebral blood supply. Each vertebral artery ascends through the neck within the transverse foramina of the cervical vertebrae C6 through C1, a protected course that reduces the risk of traumatic injury. After exiting the transverse foramen of C1, the vertebral artery follows a tortuous path, passing posteriorly around the lateral mass of C1 before piercing the dura mater and entering the cranial cavity through the foramen magnum.

At the lower border of the pons, the two vertebral arteries merge to form the basilar artery, a single midline vessel that ascends along the ventral surface of the pons. Before merging, each vertebral artery gives off several important branches, including the posterior inferior cerebellar artery (PICA) and the anterior spinal artery. The basilar artery terminates at the upper border of the pons by bifurcating into the two posterior cerebral arteries.

Major Branches of the Vertebrobasilar System

Posterior Inferior Cerebellar Artery (PICA) This is typically the largest branch of the vertebral artery and supplies the posterior and inferior portions of the cerebellum, as well as the lateral medulla. PICA occlusion produces lateral medullary syndrome (Wallenberg syndrome), characterized by ipsilateral facial pain and temperature loss, Horner syndrome, ataxia, and contralateral body pain and temperature loss.

Anterior Inferior Cerebellar Artery (AICA) Arising from the lower portion of the basilar artery, AICA supplies the anterior and inferior cerebellum and portions of the lateral pons. It also gives off the labyrinthine artery (or internal auditory artery), which supplies the inner ear. AICA occlusion can cause ipsilateral hearing loss, vertigo, facial weakness, and cerebellar signs.

Pontine Arteries Multiple small perforating arteries arise directly from the basilar artery along its course, supplying the pons. These vessels can be categorized as paramedian perforators (supplying medial structures), short circumferential branches (supplying lateral structures), and long circumferential branches (reaching more lateral and dorsal structures). The pons contains critical structures including the corticospinal and corticobulbar tracts, medial lemniscus, middle cerebellar peduncles, and various cranial nerve nuclei.

Superior Cerebellar Artery (SCA) Arising from the basilar artery just before its terminal bifurcation, the SCA supplies the superior cerebellum and portions of the midbrain. It courses around the cerebral peduncles, passing between the posterior cerebral artery superiorly and the superior cerebellar artery inferiorly. SCA territory infarction produces ipsilateral cerebellar ataxia, contralateral pain and temperature loss, and sometimes Horner syndrome.

Posterior Cerebral Arteries (PCA) The PCAs are the terminal branches of the basilar artery and supply the occipital lobes, inferior and medial temporal lobes, and portions of the thalamus and midbrain. The PCA territory includes the primary visual cortex (calcarine cortex), making PCA occlusion a common cause of homonymous hemianopsia. Each PCA gives off several important branches: the thalamoperforating arteries (supplying the thalamus), the posterior choroidal arteries (supplying the choroid plexus and thalamus), and cortical branches including the calcarine artery (visual cortex), posterior temporal branches, and parieto-occipital branches.

The Circle of Willis and Collateral Circulation

The Circle of Willis is an anastomotic ring of arteries located at the base of the brain, surrounding the optic chiasm and hypothalamus. This vascular structure represents one of the most important collateral pathways in the body, connecting the internal carotid (anterior) circulation with the vertebrobasilar (posterior) circulation. The circle provides a mechanism for maintaining cerebral perfusion even when one or more of the major feeding arteries becomes compromised.

Components of the Circle of Willis

The Circle of Willis is formed by the following vessels, arranged in a roughly hexagonal configuration:

- *Anterior cerebral arteries (ACA):* Two vessels arising from the internal carotid arteries, coursing medially
- *Anterior communicating artery:* A short vessel connecting the two anterior cerebral arteries across the midline
- *Internal carotid arteries:* The terminal portions of the ICAs contribute to the lateral aspects of the circle
- *Posterior communicating arteries:* Two vessels connecting the internal carotid arteries with the posterior cerebral arteries
- *Posterior cerebral arteries (PCA):* Two vessels arising from the basilar artery bifurcation, forming the posterior aspect of the circle

The Circle of Willis provides several clinically important collateral pathways. Blood can flow from the carotid circulation to the vertebrobasilar territory (or vice versa) through the posterior communicating arteries. The anterior communicating artery allows blood to cross from one cerebral hemisphere to the other if one internal carotid artery becomes occluded. However, anatomical variations in the circle are extremely common—only about 20–25% of individuals have a complete, symmetrical circle. Common variations include hypoplastic or absent posterior communicating arteries, asymmetric anterior cerebral arteries, and variations in the origin of the posterior cerebral arteries. These anatomical variations can affect collateral capacity and influence an individual's vulnerability to stroke.

Territorial Distribution of Major Cerebral Arteries

Understanding the territorial distribution of the major cerebral arteries is essential for localizing lesions based on clinical presentation and for interpreting neuroimaging studies. Each major artery supplies distinct cortical and subcortical regions with specific functional correlates.

Anterior Cerebral Artery Territory

The ACA supplies the medial aspects of the frontal and parietal lobes, including the superior frontal gyrus, paracentral lobule, and precuneus. This territory encompasses the motor and sensory cortices for the lower extremities and the supplementary motor area. The ACA also supplies portions of the corpus callosum through its pericallosal and callosomarginal branches. Deep perforating branches from the proximal ACA (including the recurrent artery of Heubner) supply the anterior limb of the internal capsule, head of the caudate nucleus, and portions of the putamen and anterior hypothalamus.

Clinically, ACA territory infarction typically produces contralateral leg weakness and sensory loss, with relative sparing of the upper extremity and face. Additional features may include urinary incontinence (due to involvement of the paracentral lobule), abulia or frontal lobe behavioral changes, and transcortical motor aphasia if the supplementary motor area in the dominant hemisphere is affected.

Middle Cerebral Artery Territory

The MCA has the largest territorial distribution of any cerebral artery, supplying the lateral aspects of the frontal, parietal, and temporal lobes. The MCA territory includes the primary motor cortex (precentral gyrus), primary somatosensory cortex (postcentral gyrus), and the language areas in the dominant hemisphere—Broca's area in the inferior frontal gyrus and Wernicke's area in the superior temporal gyrus. Deep penetrating branches (lenticulostriate arteries) supply the basal ganglia (caudate and putamen), most of the internal capsule, and parts of the thalamus.

MCA stroke is the most common type of ischemic stroke and produces a characteristic clinical syndrome. Complete MCA territory infarction causes contralateral hemiplegia and hemisensory loss affecting the face and upper extremity more than the lower extremity, contralateral homonymous hemianopsia, and gaze deviation toward the side of the lesion. If the dominant hemisphere is affected, global aphasia typically occurs. Involvement of the non-dominant hemisphere may cause hemineglect syndrome. Superior division MCA strokes primarily affect motor function and produce Broca's aphasia, while inferior division strokes primarily affect sensory function and produce Wernicke's aphasia and visual field deficits.

Posterior Cerebral Artery Territory

The PCA supplies the occipital lobes (including the primary visual cortex along the calcarine fissure), the inferior and medial portions of the temporal lobes (including parts of the hippocampus), and the posterior thalamus and midbrain. Perforating branches supply much of the thalamus, which serves as a critical relay station for sensory information ascending to the cortex.

PCA territory infarction most commonly produces contralateral homonymous hemianopsia with macular sparing (because the macular region of the visual cortex often receives collateral supply from the MCA). Bilateral PCA infarction can cause cortical blindness. Thalamic involvement may cause hemisensory loss, and temporal lobe involvement can produce memory deficits. Occlusion of the proximal PCA or its perforating branches can affect the midbrain, producing third nerve palsy, contralateral hemiplegia (Weber syndrome), or other complex brainstem syndromes.

Cerebellar Artery Territories

The cerebellum receives blood supply from three paired arteries, each with distinct territories:

- *PICA* supplies the posterior and inferior cerebellum and the dorsolateral medulla.
- *AICA* supplies the anterior and inferior cerebellum, flocculus, and lateral pons.
- *SCA* supplies the superior cerebellum and portions of the midbrain.

A useful anatomical landmark is the horizontal fissure of the cerebellum, which roughly demarcates the SCA territory (above) from the PICA territory (below). Cerebellar infarctions produce ipsilateral ataxia, dysmetria, and intention tremor, often accompanied by brainstem signs depending on which perforating branches are affected.

Cerebral Venous Drainage

The venous drainage of the brain differs fundamentally from the systemic venous system. Rather than draining into conventional veins with valves, cerebral blood drains into dural venous sinuses (depicted in Fig. 9.2 schematically and in Fig. 9.3 anatomically)—endothelium-lined channels within the dura mater that lack valves and therefore permit bidirectional flow under certain conditions. Understanding venous anatomy is crucial for recognizing venous thrombosis and interpreting neurosurgical procedures.

Major Dural Venous Sinuses

Superior Sagittal Sinus This large unpaired sinus runs in the midline along the superior margin of the falx cerebri, from the foramen cecum anteriorly to the internal occipital protuberance (confluence of sinuses) posteriorly. It receives blood from the superior cortical veins and communicates with the scalp veins through emissary veins. The arachnoid granulations protrude into the superior sagittal sinus, allowing cerebrospinal fluid to drain into the venous system.

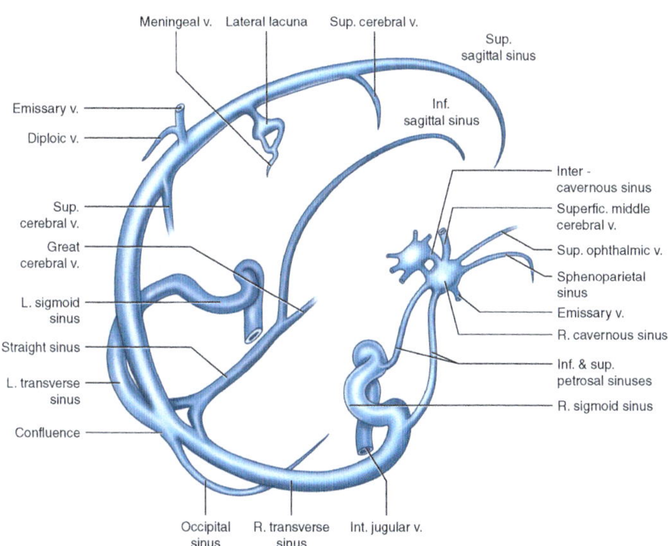

Fig. 9.2 Schematic diagram of the dural venous sinuses and cerebral veins, including the superior and inferior sagittal sinuses, straight sinus, transverse and sigmoid sinuses, cavernous sinus, petrosal sinuses, confluence of sinuses, and their connections to the internal jugular vein, illustrated from a medial perspective

Inferior Sagittal Sinus Running along the inferior-free margin of the falx cerebri, this smaller sinus drains the medial surfaces of the hemispheres and joins with the great vein of Galen to form the straight sinus.

Straight Sinus Formed by the junction of the inferior sagittal sinus and the great vein of Galen, the straight sinus courses along the junction of the falx cerebri and tentorium cerebelli, draining deep brain structures before joining the confluence of sinuses.

Transverse Sinuses These paired sinuses originate at the confluence of sinuses (torcular Herophili) and course laterally along the posterior attachment of the tentorium cerebelli toward the mastoid region. The transverse sinuses receive blood from the

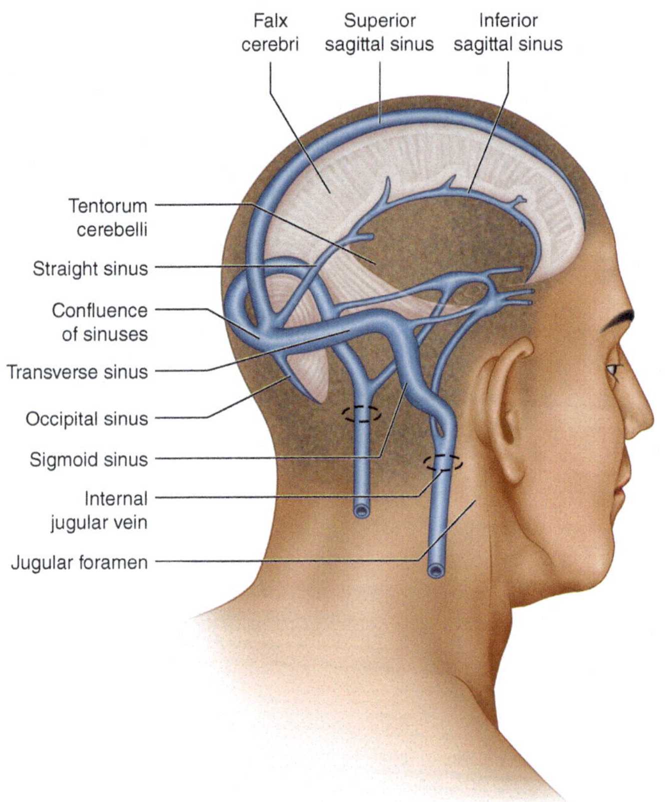

Fig. 9.3 Lateral view of the head in sagittal section showing the dural venous sinuses in situ, including the superior and inferior sagittal sinuses, straight sinus, confluence of sinuses, transverse and sigmoid sinuses, and occipital sinus, along with the falx cerebri, tentorium cerebelli, and drainage into the internal jugular vein via the jugular foramen

superior sagittal sinus, straight sinus, and various cortical and cerebellar veins.

Sigmoid Sinuses Continuing from the transverse sinuses, the sigmoid sinuses follow an S-shaped course in the posterior fossa, descending along the temporal bone before exiting the skull through the jugular foramen to become the internal jugular veins. The sigmoid sinuses also receive blood from the inferior petrosal sinuses.

Cavernous Sinuses These paired sinuses are located on either side of the sella turcica and represent perhaps the most clinically important dural sinuses due to the critical structures they contain. The internal carotid artery and abducens nerve (CN VI) pass through the sinus itself, while the oculomotor nerve (CN III), trochlear nerve (CN IV), and the ophthalmic (V1) and maxillary (V2) divisions of the trigeminal nerve course through the lateral wall of the sinus. The cavernous sinuses receive venous drainage from the orbits (via the superior and inferior ophthalmic veins), the face, and portions of the cerebral hemispheres. They drain posteriorly into the superior and inferior petrosal sinuses.

The dural venous sinuses ultimately drain into the internal jugular veins, which descend through the neck and join with the subclavian veins to form the brachiocephalic veins, eventually returning blood to the heart via the superior vena cava. Cerebral venous thrombosis can occur in any of these sinuses, producing varied clinical manifestations depending on location. Superior sagittal sinus thrombosis may cause bilateral leg weakness, seizures, and elevated intracranial pressure. Cavernous sinus thrombosis produces a characteristic syndrome of orbital pain, proptosis, ophthalmoplegia, and periorbital edema.

Deep Cerebral Venous Drainage

While the superficial cortical veins drain the cerebral cortex and subcortical white matter into the dural sinuses directly, the deep structures of the brain—including the basal ganglia, thalamus, internal capsule, and deep white matter—are drained by a separate system of deep cerebral veins that ultimately converge on the great cerebral vein of Galen (depicted in Fig. 9.4).

Internal Cerebral Veins These paired veins are the principal collectors of deep cerebral drainage. Each internal cerebral vein is formed near the interventricular foramen (of Monro) by the union of the thalamostriate vein and the septal vein. The internal cerebral veins course posteriorly within the roof of the third ventricle, running parallel to one another in the velum interpositum. They receive tributaries from the choroid plexus (choroidal veins), the thalamus, and the deep white matter before uniting posteriorly beneath the splenium of the corpus callosum to form the great cerebral vein.

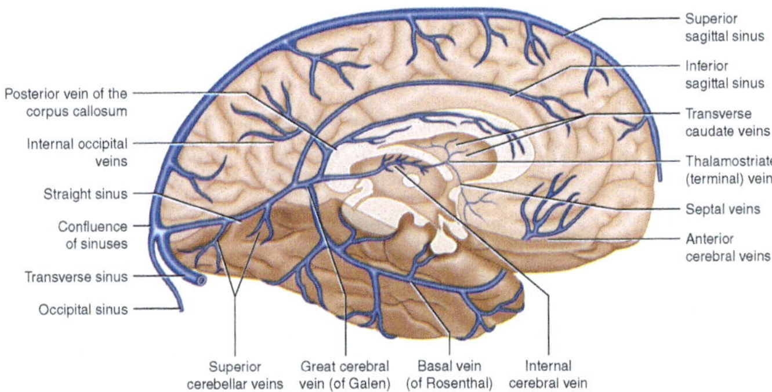

Fig. 9.4 Medial surface of the right cerebral hemisphere in sagittal section illustrating the deep cerebral venous drainage system, including the internal cerebral vein, basal vein of Rosenthal, great cerebral vein of Galen, thalamostriate and septal veins, and their relationship to the dural sinuses (superior sagittal, inferior sagittal, straight, transverse, and occipital)

Thalamostriate (Terminal) Vein This important tributary of the internal cerebral vein drains the caudate nucleus, putamen, internal capsule, and thalamus. It courses in the groove between the caudate nucleus and thalamus (the terminal sulcus) and is visible on imaging as a reliable landmark for the internal cerebral vein. Transverse caudate veins drain the body of the caudate nucleus and drain medially into the thalamostriate vein.

Septal Veins The septal veins drain the anterior horns of the lateral ventricles and the septum pellucidum, coursing posteriorly to join the internal cerebral veins at the interventricular foramen.

Basal Vein of Rosenthal This large deep vein originates near the anterior perforated substance from the union of the anterior cerebral vein and the deep middle cerebral vein. It courses posteriorly around the cerebral peduncle within the ambient cistern, collecting tributaries from the insula, inferior frontal and temporal lobes, midbrain, and the posterior perforated substance. The basal vein ultimately drains into the great cerebral vein of Galen, though it may also drain into the transverse or straight sinuses directly.

Great Cerebral Vein of Galen Formed by the union of the two internal cerebral veins beneath the splenium of the corpus callosum, the great cerebral vein of Galen is a short but critically important vessel. It also receives the basal veins of Rosenthal and the posterior vein of the corpus callosum before joining the inferior sagittal sinus to form the straight sinus. The vein of Galen is the principal conduit for deep cerebral venous drainage into the dural sinus system.

Posterior Vein of the Corpus Callosum This vein drains the posterior body and splenium of the corpus callosum, running posteriorly along the dorsal surface of the corpus callosum to drain into the great cerebral vein.

Superior Cerebellar Veins The superior surface of the cerebellum is drained by superior cerebellar veins, which course over the tentorium cerebelli and drain predominantly into the straight sinus and the great cerebral vein of Galen, thereby contributing to the deep drainage system.

The deep venous system is clinically significant for several reasons. Thrombosis of the deep cerebral veins or the vein of Galen produces a devastating syndrome of bilateral thalamic and basal ganglia infarction, often presenting with altered consciousness, coma, and poor prognosis. Arteriovenous malformations involving deep drainage carry a higher risk of hemorrhage than those draining superficially. Furthermore, the vein of Galen malformation—a distinct congenital lesion in which arterial feeders drain directly into the embryonic precursor of the great vein—presents in neonates and infants with high-output cardiac failure, hydrocephalus, and progressive neurological decline.

The Blood-Brain Barrier

The blood-brain barrier (BBB) is a highly selective permeability barrier that separates the circulating blood from the brain extracellular fluid in the central nervous system. This specialized barrier is essential for maintaining the stable extracellular environment required for proper neuronal function, protecting the brain from toxins, pathogens, and fluctuations in blood composition that occur with eating, exercise, or stress.

Structural Basis of the Blood-Brain Barrier

The BBB is formed primarily by the specialized endothelial cells that line cerebral capillaries. Unlike endothelial cells in most other organs, brain capillary endothelial cells are connected by extensive tight junctions that severely restrict paracellular (between cell) movement of molecules. These tight junctions are composed of transmembrane proteins including claudins, occludins, and junction adhesion molecules, which create a nearly impermeable seal between adjacent endothelial cells.

The barrier is further reinforced by several supporting elements. A thick basement membrane surrounds the endothelial cells, and pericytes embedded within this basement membrane provide structural support and help regulate capillary blood flow. The capillaries are ensheathed by astrocytic end-feet—processes from astrocytes that nearly completely cover the abluminal (brain-facing) surface of the capillaries. While astrocytic end-feet are not themselves part of the barrier (molecules that cross the endothelium can pass freely through the astrocytic layer), they play crucial roles in inducing and maintaining barrier properties in the endothelial cells.

Transport Across the Blood-Brain Barrier

The selective permeability of the BBB allows essential nutrients to enter the brain while excluding potentially harmful substances. Small lipophilic molecules (such as oxygen, carbon dioxide, and steroid hormones) can diffuse directly across the lipid bilayers of endothelial cells. However, most molecules require specific transport mechanisms:

- *Carrier-mediated transport:* Specific carrier proteins facilitate the movement of glucose (via GLUT1 transporters), amino acids, and other essential nutrients across the barrier.
- *Receptor-mediated transcytosis:* Larger molecules like insulin and transferrin bind to specific receptors on the luminal surface, triggering endocytosis and transport across the cell.
- *Efflux transporters:* ATP-binding cassette transporters (particularly P-glycoprotein) actively pump many drugs and toxins back into the blood, limiting their brain penetration.

Circumventricular Organs

Certain specialized brain regions called circumventricular organs lack a blood-brain barrier, allowing them to detect blood-borne signals or secrete substances directly into the circulation. These regions include the area postrema (involved in detecting toxins and triggering vomiting), the median eminence (releasing hypothalamic hormones), the organum vasculosum of the lamina terminalis (osmoreception), the subfornical organ (involved in thirst and cardiovascular regulation), the pineal gland (secreting melatonin), and the choroid plexuses (producing cerebrospinal fluid).

Clinical Significance

The blood-brain barrier presents both protection and challenges in clinical medicine. It protects the brain from most pathogens, but this protection is not absolute—certain bacteria (such as *Streptococcus pneumoniae*) and viruses can cross the barrier and cause meningitis or encephalitis. The barrier also significantly limits the delivery of therapeutic agents to the brain, with an estimated 98% of small-molecule drugs and nearly 100% of large-molecule biologics unable to cross the BBB in significant quantities. This restriction complicates the treatment of brain tumors, neurodegenerative diseases, and CNS infections. The BBB can be disrupted by inflammation, trauma, tumors, ischemia, hypertension, and certain infections. When the barrier is compromised, it can lead to vasogenic edema (accumulation of fluid in the brain parenchyma) and potentially allow entry of neurotoxic substances.

Cerebral Autoregulation and Hemodynamics

Cerebral autoregulation is the intrinsic ability of the brain's vasculature to maintain relatively constant cerebral blood flow despite changes in cerebral perfusion pressure. This mechanism is essential because neurons have high metabolic demands and virtually no energy reserves—interruption of blood flow for even a few seconds causes loss of consciousness, and a few minutes can cause irreversible injury.

Mechanisms of Autoregulation

Cerebral autoregulation operates primarily through myogenic and metabolic mechanisms. The myogenic response involves the intrinsic property of smooth muscle in arteriolar walls to contract when stretched (by increased pressure) and relax when pressure decreases. This mechanism provides rapid adjustments in vessel diameter that counteract pressure changes. The metabolic mechanism involves local release of vasoactive substances in response to tissue needs. When neuronal activity increases, the resulting elevation in carbon dioxide, adenosine, and hydrogen ions, combined with decreased oxygen, causes vasodilation and increased local blood flow. Conversely, reduced metabolic demand leads to vasoconstriction.

Under normal conditions, autoregulation maintains constant cerebral blood flow across a mean arterial pressure range of approximately 60–150 mmHg. Below this range, cerebral blood flow decreases linearly with pressure, leading to ischemia. Above this range, autoregulation fails and excessive perfusion pressure can disrupt the blood-brain barrier, causing hypertensive encephalopathy.

Factors Affecting Cerebral Blood Flow

Several physiological factors significantly influence cerebral blood flow:

- *PaCO2:* Carbon dioxide is the most potent regulator of cerebral blood flow. Hypercapnia causes cerebral vasodilation and increased flow, while hypocapnia causes vasoconstriction and decreased flow. For every 1 mmHg change in PaCO2, cerebral blood flow changes by approximately 3–4%.

- *PaO2:* Oxygen tension has less influence on cerebral blood flow under normal conditions, but severe hypoxemia (PaO2 < 50 mmHg) triggers significant vasodilation.
- *Neural Activity:* Increased neuronal activity leads to increased local blood flow through metabolic coupling (neurovascular coupling). This principle underlies functional MRI, which detects local changes in blood oxygenation related to neural activity.
- *Autonomic Innervation:* Though less important than metabolic factors, sympathetic innervation can cause some vasoconstriction, while parasympathetic and nitrergic innervation cause vasodilation.

Clinical Implications

Autoregulation can be impaired in various pathological conditions, including acute stroke, traumatic brain injury, subarachnoid hemorrhage, and severe hypertension. When autoregulation fails, cerebral blood flow becomes directly dependent on blood pressure, making the brain vulnerable to both hypoperfusion and hyperperfusion injuries. In ischemic stroke, the autoregulatory curve may be shifted rightward, requiring higher blood pressures to maintain adequate flow—this is why permissive hypertension is often appropriate in acute ischemic stroke. Understanding autoregulation is also crucial for managing patients with increased intracranial pressure, where maintaining adequate cerebral perfusion pressure (mean arterial pressure minus intracranial pressure) is essential for preventing secondary ischemic injury.

Blood Supply to the Spinal Cord

The blood supply to the spinal cord is more tenuous than the brain's blood supply, with watershed zones particularly vulnerable to ischemia. Understanding spinal vascular anatomy is critical for recognizing spinal cord infarction syndromes and for surgical planning in procedures involving the aorta or spine.

Arterial Supply to the Spinal Cord

Anterior Spinal Artery The anterior spinal artery is formed by the fusion of two branches from the vertebral arteries at the level of the foramen magnum. This single midline vessel descends along the anterior surface of the spinal cord in the anterior median fissure, extending the entire length of the cord to the conus medullaris. The anterior spinal artery supplies the anterior two-thirds of the spinal cord, including the anterior horns (motor neurons), the lateral corticospinal tracts, and the spinothalamic tracts (pain and temperature pathways). The single anterior spinal artery makes the anterior spinal cord particularly vulnerable to ischemia, as there is limited collateral circulation.

Posterior Spinal Arteries Unlike the single anterior spinal artery, there are two posterior spinal arteries that originate either directly from the vertebral arteries or from the posterior inferior cerebellar arteries. These paired arteries descend along the posterolateral surface of the spinal cord, medial to the dorsal nerve roots. The posterior spinal arteries supply the posterior one-third of the spinal cord, including the dorsal columns (carrying proprioception, vibration, and fine touch) and the dorsal horns. The dual supply provides better collateral circulation to the posterior cord.

Segmental and Radicular Arteries The anterior and posterior spinal arteries receive supplementary blood supply from segmental arteries arising from the aorta (in the thoracic and lumbar regions) or from vertebral, deep cervical, and intercostal arteries. These segmental arteries give off radicular arteries that follow the nerve roots through the intervertebral foramina to reach the spinal cord. Most radicular arteries are small and supply only the nerve roots, but several larger radiculomedullary arteries penetrate to the spinal cord surface and reinforce the longitudinal spinal arteries.

Artery of Adamkiewicz The artery of Adamkiewicz (arteria radicularis magna) is the largest anterior radiculomedullary artery and provides critical blood supply to the lower thoracic and lumbar spinal cord. It typically arises from the aorta on the left side, usually between T8 and L1 (most commonly at T9-T11), though its level of origin is quite variable. The artery of Adamkiewicz ascends with a nerve root to reach the anterior spinal artery, which it reinforces substantially. The dependence of the thoracolumbar cord on this single large feeding vessel creates a watershed zone in the mid-thoracic region (approximately T4-T8), which is vulnerable to ischemia during hypotension or aortic surgery.

Intrinsic Vascular Supply

From the anterior and posterior spinal arteries, small penetrating arteries enter the spinal cord parenchyma. Central (sulcal) arteries arise alternately from either side of the anterior spinal artery, penetrate the anterior median fissure, and supply the anterior and central portions of the cord. These vessels supply the gray matter of the anterior horns and the white matter tracts in the anterior and lateral columns. The posterior spinal arteries give off pial plexus branches that form an anastomotic network on the cord surface before penetrating to supply the posterior white matter columns and dorsal horns. A peripheral arterial network (vasocorona) around the cord surface receives contributions from both anterior and posterior systems, providing some collateral circulation.

Venous Drainage of the Spinal Cord

Venous drainage follows a pattern roughly reciprocal to the arterial supply. Six small longitudinal venous channels—anterior and posterior median veins, and paired anterolateral and posterolateral veins—drain into an extensive internal vertebral venous plexus (epidural venous plexus) that lies within the vertebral canal but outside the dura mater. This valveless plexus communicates freely with segmental veins that drain into the systemic venous system (azygos, hemiazygos, and lumbar veins). The absence of valves means blood flow direction can reverse, which may allow metastatic tumor cells to spread to the vertebral column (Batson's plexus).

Clinical Syndromes of Spinal Cord Ischemia

Anterior Spinal Artery Syndrome Occlusion of the anterior spinal artery produces a characteristic syndrome reflecting damage to structures in the anterior two-thirds of the cord. Patients develop acute paraplegia or quadriplegia (depending on the level of infarction) due to involvement of the anterior horn motor neurons and corticospinal tracts. Loss of pain and temperature sensation occurs bilaterally below the lesion due to spinothalamic tract involvement. Critically, proprioception, vibration sense, and fine discriminative touch are preserved because the dorsal columns are supplied by the posterior spinal arteries. Autonomic dysfunction may occur, including neurogenic bladder and bowel dysfunction. This syndrome can result from aortic surgery, aortic dissection, severe hypotension, atherosclerosis, or thromboembolism.

Posterior Spinal Artery Syndrome Isolated posterior spinal artery infarction is rare due to the dual arterial supply and better collateral circulation. When it occurs, it produces loss of proprioception, vibration sense, and fine touch below the level of the lesion, with preserved motor function and pain/temperature sensation. Patients may develop sensory ataxia due to loss of proprioceptive feedback.

Cauda Equina Syndrome While not strictly a vascular syndrome, cauda equina syndrome results from compression or ischemia of the lumbosacral nerve roots below the conus medullaris. The syndrome presents with low back pain, bilateral leg weakness (often asymmetric), saddle anesthesia (loss of sensation in the perineal region), and bladder/bowel dysfunction (including urinary retention and fecal incontinence). This is a neurological emergency requiring urgent decompression to prevent permanent dysfunction.

Clinical Stroke Syndromes

Recognition of stroke syndromes based on vascular territories is essential for clinical diagnosis, acute management decisions, and prognostication. The clinical presentation reflects both the location and extent of ischemia.

Anterior Circulation Strokes

Left MCA Superior Division Stroke Produces Broca's aphasia (non-fluent aphasia with preserved comprehension), right arm and facial weakness (face and arm regions of motor cortex), and possible right-sided sensory loss. The leg is typically spared because its representation is in the ACA territory.

Left MCA Inferior Division Stroke Results in Wernicke's aphasia (fluent aphasia with impaired comprehension), right superior quadrantanopsia (due to involvement of Meyer's loop—the temporal lobe portion of the optic radiations), and right arm/facial sensory loss affecting the somatosensory cortex.

Right MCA Superior Division Stroke Causes left arm and facial weakness without aphasia (in right-handed individuals) and may produce left-sided neglect if parietal regions are involved.

Right MCA Inferior Division Stroke Produces left hemineglect syndrome (neglect of the left side of space), left superior quadrantanopsia, and left arm/facial sensory deficits.

ACA Territory Strokes Left ACA infarction causes right leg weakness and sensory loss, while right ACA infarction causes left leg weakness and sensory loss. Additional features may include abulia (apathy and reduced motivation), urinary incontinence, and grasp reflexes.

Posterior Circulation Strokes

PCA Territory Strokes Left PCA infarction produces right homonymous hemianopsia (often with macular sparing), while right PCA infarction causes left homonymous hemianopsia. Bilateral PCA infarction can cause cortical blindness with preserved pupillary reflexes. If the infarct involves the temporal lobe, memory deficits may occur.

Brainstem Strokes Brainstem infarctions produce complex syndromes often involving cranial nerve deficits ipsilateral to the lesion combined with long tract signs contralateral to the lesion. Lateral medullary syndrome (Wallenberg syndrome from PICA occlusion) presents with ipsilateral facial pain/temperature loss, Horner syndrome, ataxia, dysphagia, and dysarthria, combined with contralateral body pain/temperature loss. Medial medullary syndrome produces ipsilateral tongue weakness and contralateral hemiparesis with proprioceptive loss. Locked-in syndrome results from bilateral ventral pontine infarction, leaving patients quadriplegic and mute but conscious, with preserved vertical eye movements.

Deep Structure Strokes

Small vessel occlusions affecting deep penetrating arteries produce lacunar infarcts with characteristic syndromes:

- *Lenticulostriate artery occlusion*: Affects the caudate nucleus and putamen, potentially causing pure motor hemiparesis, dysarthria-clumsy hand syndrome, or choreoathetosis
- *Recurrent artery of Heubner occlusion*: Damages the nucleus accumbens and anterior caudate head
- *Anterior choroidal artery occlusion*: Affects the globus pallidus and posterior limb of internal capsule, causing contralateral hemiplegia, hemisensory loss, and hemianopsia
- *Thalamoperforating artery occlusion*: Produces pure sensory stroke with contralateral hemisensory loss
- *Thalamogeniculate artery occlusion*: Affects the ventral thalamus, causing sensory deficits and sometimes thalamic pain syndrome
- *Posterior choroidal artery occlusion*: Involves the medial dorsal thalamus, potentially causing memory deficits and behavioral changes

Cerebral Herniation

The rigid skull, while protective, creates a closed compartment with fixed volume. Under normal circumstances, the brain parenchyma, cerebrospinal fluid, and cerebral blood volume exist in equilibrium within this space—a relationship described by the Monro-Kellie doctrine. When a space-occupying lesion develops, whether from hematoma, tumor, edema, or abscess, compensatory mechanisms initially buffer the rise in intracranial pressure. Once these mechanisms are exhausted, pressure differentials develop between compartments, and brain tissue is forced through anatomical openings in a process termed cerebral herniation. Figure 9.5 illustrates the six major herniation syndromes that can result from such pressure gradients.

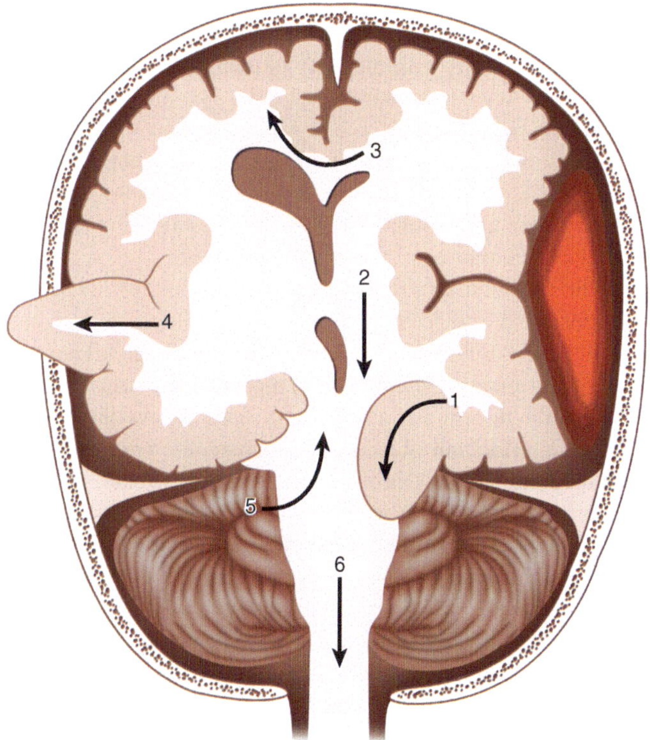

Fig. 9.5 Coronal section of the brain illustrating the six major types of cerebral herniation caused by a right-sided mass lesion (shown in red). Numbered arrows indicate (1) uncal herniation, in which the medial temporal lobe is displaced over the tentorial edge compressing the midbrain; (2) central (transtentorial) herniation, with downward displacement of the diencephalon through the tentorial notch; (3) cingulate (subfalcine) herniation, in which the cingulate gyrus is forced under the falx cerebri toward the contralateral hemisphere; (4) transcalvarial herniation, in which brain tissue herniates through a skull defect; (5) upward cerebellar/transtentorial herniation, with upward displacement of the cerebellum through the tentorial notch; and (6) downward cerebellar (tonsillar) herniation, in which the cerebellar tonsils are displaced through the foramen magnum

Cingulate (subfalcine) herniation is the most common form and occurs when a unilateral hemispheric mass displaces the cingulate gyrus medially and inferiorly beneath the free edge of the falx cerebri toward the contralateral side. The anterior cerebral artery and its branches may be compressed against the falx, risking infarction of the medial frontal and parietal cortex. Contralateral leg weakness is the characteristic clinical manifestation. Subfalcine herniation frequently precedes and contributes to transtentorial herniation as the process progresses.

Central (transtentorial) herniation results from downward displacement of the diencephalon and medial temporal structures through the tentorial notch, typically caused by large bilateral or midline supratentorial lesions. The process compresses the midbrain, distorts the reticular activating system, and produces a rostrocaudal deterioration of neurological function. Clinically, this manifests as progressive impairment of consciousness, Cheyne-Stokes respiration, small reactive pupils, and decorticate then decerebrate posturing as the brainstem is sequentially compressed from above downward.

Uncal herniation is the most clinically recognizable herniation syndrome. A unilateral temporal lobe mass—most commonly an extradural or subdural hematoma—pushes the medial temporal lobe (the uncus and parahippocampal gyrus) over the free edge of the tentorium cerebelli. The herniating uncus compresses the ipsilateral oculomotor nerve (CN III) against the posterior communicating artery or the tentorial edge, producing the classic early sign of a fixed, dilated ipsilateral pupil due to disruption of parasympathetic pupillomotor fibers that travel on the outer surface of CN III. As herniation progresses, the ipsilateral cerebral peduncle is compressed, causing contralateral hemiplegia. In approximately 25% of cases, the contralateral peduncle is compressed against the opposite tentorial edge (Kernohan's notch), producing an ipsilateral hemiplegia that constitutes a false localizing sign.

Transcalvarial herniation occurs when brain tissue extrudes through a defect in the skull, either through a fracture site or a surgical craniotomy opening. This is most commonly encountered postoperatively or following traumatic injury and represents the only form of herniation in which brain tissue exits the intracranial compartment entirely.

Upward cerebellar (transtentorial) herniation occurs when a posterior fossa mass—such as a cerebellar hematoma, abscess, or tumor—generates sufficient upward pressure to displace the superior vermis and cerebellar hemispheres upward through the tentorial notch. This compresses the midbrain from below and may occlude the cerebral aqueduct, causing obstructive hydrocephalus. The superior cerebellar arteries and posterior cerebral arteries may be compromised, and the tectal plate is typically compressed, producing upgaze palsy.

Downward cerebellar (tonsillar) herniation represents the most immediately life-threatening herniation syndrome. Raised pressure in the posterior fossa—or global elevation of intracranial pressure—forces the cerebellar tonsils downward through the foramen magnum, compressing the medulla oblongata. Since the medulla contains the vital centers for cardiovascular and respiratory control, tonsillar herniation rapidly produces cardiorespiratory arrest. This is the pathological basis for the danger of performing lumbar puncture in the presence of raised intracranial pressure, as sudden reduction in spinal CSF pressure can precipitate acute downward herniation.

Intracranial Hemorrhage

Bleeding within or around the brain can occur in several anatomically distinct compartments, each with characteristic clinical presentations, etiologies, and management strategies. Figure 9.6 illustrates the six principal types of intracranial hemorrhage in axial section, demonstrating their spatial relationships to the brain parenchyma and its meningeal coverings.

Extradural (epidural) hemorrhage occurs in the potential space between the inner surface of the skull and the outer (periosteal) layer of the dura mater. This space does not exist under normal conditions—the dura is tightly adherent to the skull—but is created by the stripping force of an expanding hematoma, most commonly arterial in origin. The classic etiology is rupture of the

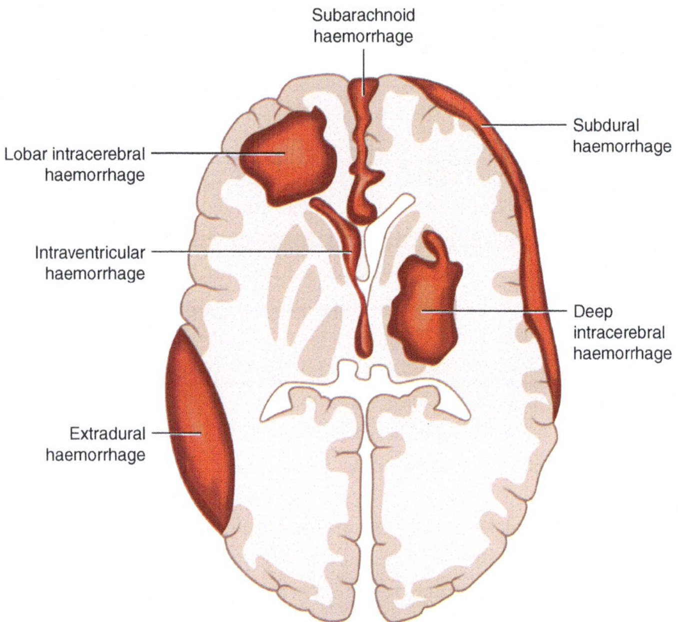

Fig. 9.6 Axial section of the brain depicting the anatomical locations of the major types of intracranial hemorrhage, including subarachnoid, subdural, extradural, lobar intracerebral, deep intracerebral, and intraventricular hemorrhage

middle meningeal artery following a temporal bone fracture, though venous sources from dural sinuses or diploic veins can also be responsible. On imaging, the extradural hematoma appears as a biconvex (lenticular) hyperdense collection, as the hematoma is limited by the cranial sutures where the dura is most firmly attached. The characteristic clinical history is of a lucid interval following initial head injury—brief loss of consciousness, apparent recovery, then rapid neurological deterioration—though this sequence occurs in only a minority of cases. Extradural hematoma is a neurosurgical emergency: the arterial bleeding is under high pressure and expands rapidly, and without prompt surgical evacuation, transtentorial herniation and death follow.

Subdural hemorrhage occupies the space between the inner layer of the dura mater and the arachnoid membrane. Unlike the extradural space, the subdural space is a real potential space traversed by bridging veins that connect the cortical surface to the dural sinuses. These veins are vulnerable to shearing forces during acceleration-deceleration head injury, particularly in the elderly and in those with cerebral atrophy, where the greater distance between cortex and dura places increased tension on the bridging veins. Subdural hematomas are therefore venous in origin, expand more slowly than extradural collections, and characteristically appear as crescent-shaped collections that follow the contour of the brain surface, unconstrained by suture lines. They are classified as acute (presenting within 72 hours), subacute (3–21 days), or chronic (beyond 21 days). Chronic subdural hematomas are particularly common in the elderly and may present insidiously with cognitive decline, headache, or fluctuating neurological deficit weeks after a seemingly trivial injury.

Subarachnoid hemorrhage refers to bleeding into the subarachnoid space—the CSF-filled compartment between the arachnoid and pia mater. Spontaneous (non-traumatic) subarachnoid hemorrhage is most commonly caused by rupture of an intracranial aneurysm, typically at branch points of the circle of Willis. The sudden release of arterial blood into the subarachnoid space under systemic pressure produces the hallmark symptom of a sudden-onset, severe headache—often described by patients as the worst headache of their life. Blood disperses rapidly through the CSF pathways, accounting for the global distribution of symptoms including meningism, photophobia, and loss of consciousness. Complications include rebleeding, cerebral vasospasm (leading to delayed ischemic neurological deficit), obstructive or communicating hydrocephalus from blockage of CSF pathways by blood, and hyponatremia from cerebral salt wasting.

Lobar intracerebral hemorrhage refers to hematomas within the cerebral lobes—the frontal, parietal, temporal, or occipital regions—typically involving the subcortical white matter. In younger patients, lobar hemorrhage is often associated with vascular malformations, coagulopathy, or drug use (particularly cocaine and amphetamines). In older patients, cerebral amyloid angiopathy—the deposition of amyloid protein in the walls of cortical and leptomeningeal vessels, rendering them fragile—is the dominant etiology and characteristically produces recurrent lobar hemorrhages at different sites over time. Lobar hemorrhages tend to be larger than deep hemorrhages and carry significant mass effect and risk of cortical spread into the subarachnoid space.

Deep intracerebral hemorrhage arises from rupture of small perforating arteries deep within the brain substance, most commonly at sites including the putamen, thalamus, caudate nucleus, pons, and cerebellum. Chronic hypertension is the dominant etiology, causing lipohyalinosis and Charcot-Bouchard microaneurysm formation in the lenticulostriate and thalamoperforating vessels. Putaminal hemorrhage—the most common site—classically presents with contralateral hemiplegia, hemisensory loss, and homonymous hemianopia, with conjugate eye deviation toward the side of the lesion. Thalamic hemorrhage may produce a characteristic downward and inward gaze deviation. Pontine hemorrhage carries a particularly poor prognosis, with rapid onset of coma, quadriplegia, and pinpoint pupils from damage to the pontine tegmentum. Cerebellar hemorrhage presents with sudden onset of severe headache, vomiting, truncal ataxia, and inability to walk, and requires urgent surgical consideration as the posterior fossa is a closed compartment with little capacity to accommodate expanding hematoma.

Intraventricular hemorrhage refers to blood within the ventricular system. It may occur as a primary event, most commonly from rupture of a subependymal arteriovenous malformation or cavernoma adjacent to the ventricle, or as a secondary extension of a parenchymal hemorrhage—particularly deep intracerebral hemorrhage—into the ventricular cavity. Blood within the ventricles can obstruct CSF flow at the aqueduct or fourth ventricular outlets, producing acute obstructive hydrocephalus that may require emergency external ventricular drainage. The presence of intraventricular hemorrhage significantly worsens the prognosis of intracerebral hemorrhage and is an independent predictor of mortality.

Conclusion

The vascular supply to the central nervous system represents a masterpiece of biological engineering, providing the enormous metabolic demands of neural tissue while maintaining remarkable stability through autoregulation and collateral pathways. Understanding the anatomy and physiology of cerebrovascular circulation is fundamental to clinical neurology and neurosurgery. The territorial organization of major arteries creates predictable clinical syndromes that guide diagnosis and localization. The Circle of Willis provides crucial collateral circulation, though its anatomical variations influence individual vulnerability to vascular occlusion. The blood-brain barrier maintains the specialized neuronal environment but complicates drug delivery. Autoregulatory mechanisms normally maintain constant cerebral perfusion across a wide range of blood pressures, but these mechanisms can fail in pathological states. The spinal cord's more tenuous blood supply creates watershed zones vulnerable to ischemia, particularly in the mid-thoracic region. Clinical recognition of stroke syndromes—whether affecting anterior circulation, posterior circulation, deep structures, or the spinal cord—enables rapid diagnosis and appropriate intervention. As medical students and residents develop expertise in neuroanatomy, this vascular framework provides essential context for understanding neurological disease, interpreting neuroimaging, and delivering optimal patient care.

Neurodevelopment 10

Neural Tube Formation and Early Development

The development of the nervous system begins with the formation of the neural tube through two distinct but complementary processes: primary and secondary neurulation. Understanding these processes is fundamental to comprehending both normal neuroanatomy and the pathophysiology of neural tube defects.

Primary Neurulation

Primary neurulation involves the transformation of the neural plate, a specialized region of ectodermal tissue, into the neural tube. This process begins when the neural plate ectoderm undergoes invagination, creating bilateral neural folds along the rostral-caudal axis of the embryo. These neural folds progressively elevate and converge toward the dorsal midline, eventually fusing to form the neural tube. This structure will give rise to the brain and the majority of the spinal cord. The precise coordination of cell shape changes, tissue movements, and molecular signaling required for primary neurulation represents one of the earliest and most critical events in nervous system development.

V. Yanamadala, *Essential Neuroanatomy*,
https://doi.org/10.1007/978-3-032-26877-8_10

Secondary Neurulation

Secondary neurulation occurs at the caudal end of the developing embryo and involves a distinctly different cellular mechanism compared to primary neurulation. In this process, mesenchymal cells in the tail bud region undergo condensation and coalescence to form a solid rod of tissue. Subsequently, this cellular rod undergoes cavitation, creating a lumen that becomes continuous with the neural tube formed through primary neurulation. Secondary neurulation is responsible for forming the most caudal portions of the spinal cord, approximately corresponding to the sacral and coccygeal segments.

Neural Tube Closure

The final and perhaps most clinically significant step in primary neurulation is neural tube closure, which occurs between days 25 and 27 of human embryonic development. Closure proceeds bidirectionally from multiple closure sites, with the anterior neuropore closing slightly before the posterior neuropore. The precise timing and spatial coordination of neural tube closure is critical, as failures at different sites along the neuraxis result in distinct clinical entities.

Neural Tube Defects

Neural tube defects represent some of the most common congenital malformations affecting the central nervous system, with an incidence of approximately 1 in 1000 live births. The clinical presentation and severity of these defects correlate directly with the location and extent of the closure failure. Anencephaly results from failure of anterior neural tube closure, leading to absence of major portions of the brain and skull. This condition is incompatible with life. Craniorachischisis represents a more severe posterior closure defect, resulting in an open neural tube along much of the spinal cord. Spina bifida cystica involves a far posterior closure defect, typically affecting the lumbosacral region, and is characterized by herniation of meninges and neural tissue through a vertebral defect. In contrast, spina bifida occulta results from defects in secondary neurulation and typically presents as a relatively benign vertebral arch defect without herniation of neural contents. The recognition that folic acid supplementation during the periconceptional period significantly reduces the incidence of neural tube defects has been one of the major public health achievements in preventive medicine.

Neural Progenitor Populations and Regional Specification

Following neural tube closure, the developing nervous system contains distinct populations of neural progenitors that give rise to the diverse array of neurons and glial cells found in the mature nervous system. Four principal sources of neural progenitors have been identified: the ventricular zone, the subventricular zone, the rhombic lip, and the neural crest.

The ventricular zone lines the central canal of the neural tube and represents the primary germinal zone where most neurons are generated. Adjacent to this is the subventricular zone, which becomes increasingly prominent as development proceeds and serves as a source of both neurons and glial cells. The rhombic lip, located at the dorsal margin of the developing hindbrain, gives rise to specific neuronal populations including cerebellar granule cells. The neural crest, discussed in detail below, represents a unique population of migratory cells with remarkable developmental potential.

Spinal Cord Organization

The developing spinal cord exhibits a characteristic three-zone organization that reflects the sequential stages of neuronal differentiation and migration. The ventricular zone, as mentioned above, contains the proliferative neural progenitors. The mantle zone, located peripheral to the ventricular zone, contains the cell bodies of postmitotic neurons that have migrated away from the ventricular surface. Finally, the marginal zone forms the outermost layer and contains the axons of developing neurons; this layer will eventually become the white matter of the mature spinal cord. This orderly laminar organization provides an elegant framework for understanding how complex neural circuits are assembled during development.

The Neural Crest

The neural crest represents a truly remarkable population of cells that has been described as the fourth germ layer due to its extensive contribution to diverse tissues throughout the body. Neural crest cells arise from the dorsal neural tube at the boundary between the epidermis and the neural plate. Their induction requires bone morphogenetic proteins (BMPs) and involves a precisely orchestrated cascade of transcription factors that confer neural crest identity.

Neural crest cells exhibit striking regional differences in their developmental potential and migratory behavior. At cranial levels, neural crest cells give rise to a wide array of tissues in the face and head, including craniofacial bones, cartilage, connective tissue, and specific neuronal populations. The trunk neural crest serves as the major source for neurons and supporting cells of the peripheral nervous system, including dorsal root ganglia neurons, sympathetic neurons, and Schwann cells. Neural crest cells arising from the vagal and sacral regions undertake extensive migrations to populate the enteric nervous system throughout the gastrointestinal tract.

Waardenburg syndrome exemplifies the clinical consequences of neural crest defects. This condition, caused by mutations in PAX3 and other genes involved in neural crest development, presents with a constellation of findings including sensorineural hearing loss, partial albinism, Hirschsprung disease (absence of enteric ganglia), and characteristic facial dysmorphology. The diverse manifestations of this syndrome reflect the multiple tissues and cell types derived from the neural crest.

PAX Genes and Dorsal-Ventral Patterning

The establishment of cellular identity along the dorsal-ventral axis of the neural tube depends on the expression of PAX genes, which encode transcription factors activated by specific morphogens. PAX3 is critical for dorsal (alar plate) differentiation, while PAX6 drives ventral (basal plate) differentiation. These transcription factors orchestrate the expression of downstream genes that determine neuronal subtype identity. The rhombic lip, expressing specific transcription factors under PAX gene control, serves as the source of cerebellar granule cells, the most numerous neurons in the entire nervous system.

Axonal Guidance Mechanisms

The formation of functional neural circuits requires that developing axons navigate through the complex three-dimensional environment of the embryo to reach their appropriate targets. This remarkable feat of cellular navigation is accomplished through the growth cone, a specialized structure at the tip of the growing axon that is capable of sensing and responding to multiple guidance cues in the environment. Four major families of guidance molecules have been identified: netrins, semaphorins, slits, and ephrins.

Netrins

Netrins are bifunctional guidance molecules that can serve as either attractants or repellents, depending on the receptors expressed by the responding neuron. When netrins bind to DCC (deleted in colon cancer) or neogenin receptors, they function as chemoattractants, drawing axons toward the source of netrin. In contrast, when netrins bind to Unc5a receptors, they function as chemorepellents. This dual functionality allows netrin gradients to simultaneously attract certain axons while repelling others, enabling the formation of complex axonal trajectories.

Semaphorins

Semaphorins represent a large family of secreted and membrane-bound guidance molecules that generally function as chemorepellents. They bind to receptors of the neuropilin and plexin families to mediate inhibitory guidance signals. A particularly elegant example of semaphorin function is seen in the guidance of dorsal root ganglion neurons. Semaphorin 3A (Sema3A) is produced in a concentration gradient in the ventral neural tube. Only nociceptive neurons express neuropilin and plexin receptors and are therefore repelled by Sema3A, causing them to project dorsally. In contrast, neurons of the ventral spinocerebellar tract do not express these receptors and are therefore insensitive to Sema3A, allowing them to project ventrally. This differential receptor expression creates distinct projection patterns from a common population of dorsal root ganglion neurons.

Slits and Robo Receptors

Slits are large secreted proteins that bind to Robo (Roundabout) receptors to mediate axon guidance. The Slit-Robo system plays a particularly important role in guiding commissural axons across the midline. Slit proteins bind to Robo1 and Robo2 receptors and function as inhibitory signals, preventing axons from crossing the midline inappropriately. However, Robo3 functions as an inhibitor of Robo1 and Robo2, effectively silencing the repulsive response to Slit. This complex receptor system allows precise control over midline crossing behavior.

Ephrins and Topographic Mapping

Ephrins and their Eph receptors (EphA and EphB receptor tyrosine kinases) play a crucial role in establishing topographic maps, particularly in the visual system. The chemoaffinity hypothesis, proposed by Roger Sperry based on his elegant experiments with regenerating optic nerves in amphibians, posited that permanent chemical cues must be present in target tissues and recognized by regenerating axons. Subsequent molecular studies confirmed this hypothesis and identified ephrins as key molecules in establishing gradients in the optic tectum.

In the developing visual system, Eph receptors are expressed at high levels in temporal retinal neurons and at low levels in nasal neurons. Conversely, ephrin ligands are expressed at high levels in the posterior tectum and at low levels in the anterior tectum. This complementary gradient system results in temporal retinal axons, which express high levels of Eph receptors, projecting to the anterior tectum where ephrin levels are low. This elegant molecular mechanism ensures that the topographic organization of the retina is preserved in its central projections, forming the basis for organized visual representations in the brain.

Switching Guidance Responses at the Midline

One of the most sophisticated aspects of axon guidance is the ability of growth cones to switch their responses to guidance cues as they navigate through different regions. This is particularly evident in commissural axons that must cross the midline. These axons are initially attracted to the midline by netrin but must then be repelled from the midline after crossing to prevent recrossing.

This switching behavior depends on changes in intracellular second messenger concentrations, particularly cyclic AMP (cAMP) and cyclic GMP (cGMP). Slit decreases cAMP levels in the growth cone, which causes netrin signaling to switch from attractive to repulsive. Additionally, Robo3/Rig1, a receptor that is mutated in horizontal gaze palsy with progressive scoliosis

(HGPPS), is expressed until the neuron reaches the midline. After crossing, Robo3 expression ceases, allowing the neuron to respond to Slit signaling from the midline. Furthermore, EphA2 receptors are synthesized only after the axon crosses the midline, making the neuron newly responsive to inhibitory ephrin signals that prevent recrossing. This multi-layered regulatory system ensures reliable unidirectional midline crossing.

Dendritic Guidance

While much attention has focused on axonal guidance, dendrites must also navigate to appropriate regions to receive synaptic inputs. Interestingly, dendrites can respond differently to the same guidance cues that direct axons. DSCAM (Down syndrome cell adhesion molecule), which serves as a netrin receptor, mediates self-inhibition to prevent dendrites from the same neuron from covering the same territory, thereby promoting tiling in retinal and somatosensory systems.

Semaphorin 3A, which repels axons expressing neuropilin receptors, actually attracts dendrites. This opposite response occurs because cGMP levels are higher in dendrites compared to axons, altering the downstream signaling cascades activated by neuropilin binding. This example illustrates how the same extracellular signal can produce different cellular responses depending on the intracellular signaling context.

Morphogen Signaling in Neural Development

Morphogens are inductive signals capable of directing different cell fates at different concentration thresholds. This concept, first proposed by Lewis Wolpert in his French flag model, has proven fundamental to understanding pattern formation throughout development. In the nervous system, Sonic Hedgehog (SHH) and bone morphogenetic proteins (BMPs) serve as the primary morphogens controlling dorsal-ventral patterning and cellular differentiation.

Sonic Hedgehog Signaling

Sonic Hedgehog represents one of the most intensively studied morphogens in developmental biology. SHH is synthesized as an inactive precursor that undergoes a remarkable process of autocatalytic cleavage and lipid modification. The protein possesses intrinsic serine protease activity in its C-terminal domain, which cleaves the precursor protein. During this cleavage reaction, a cholesterol molecule is covalently attached to the N-terminal signaling domain. This cholesterol modification serves to anchor the active SHH protein in the cell membrane of floor plate cells where it is synthesized.

The cholesterol anchor is crucial for establishing an appropriate SHH concentration gradient. Because cholesterol has a very low diffusion coefficient in the aqueous extracellular environment, only small quantities of SHH can diffuse away from the floor plate. This creates a steep concentration gradient from the ventral floor plate to the dorsal midline. Different neuronal subtypes are specified by different SHH concentration thresholds, with ventral-most neurons requiring the highest SHH concentrations and progressively more dorsal neurons requiring lower concentrations. This elegant mechanism allows a single signaling molecule to specify multiple distinct cell fates along the dorsal-ventral axis.

Neurotrophin Signaling and Neuronal Survival

During nervous system development, far more neurons are initially generated than will survive to maturity. This overproduction followed by selective death represents a fundamental strategy for matching neuronal numbers to target tissue size and for eliminating neurons that have made inappropriate connections. Target tissues secrete neurotrophic factors, including nerve growth factor (NGF), brain-derived neurotrophic factor (BDNF), and neurotrophin-3 (NT3), which promote the survival of neurons whose axons successfully reach appropriate targets.

The Signaling Endosome Model

How do target-derived neurotrophins, which bind to receptors on axon terminals that may be located meters away from the cell body, influence nuclear gene expression and cell survival? The signaling endosome model provides an elegant solution to this problem. According to this model, neurotrophins bound to their Trk receptors are internalized into signaling endosomes at the axon terminal. These endosomes are then transported retrograde to the cell body via dynein motor proteins and the associated protein dynactin. The signaling complex remains active during this journey and activates survival pathways upon arrival at the cell body.

Neurotrophin-Receptor Pairs

Each neurotrophin exhibits preferential binding to specific Trk receptors, although some promiscuity exists at higher ligand concentrations. NGF binds to TrkA, which is expressed in nociceptive neurons, sympathetic neurons, and cholinergic neurons. Mutations in TrkA cause congenital insensitivity to pain with anhidrosis (CIPA syndrome), characterized by inability to perceive pain, absent sweating, and mental retardation. BDNF binds to TrkB, which is expressed in many neuronal types throughout the nervous system. Mutations in BDNF cause obesity, hyperphagia, and cognitive dysfunction. NT3 binds preferentially to TrkC, although it can also activate TrkA and TrkB at high concentrations. NT4, another member of the neurotrophin family, also binds to TrkB.

Trk Receptor Signaling Pathways

Activation of Trk receptors initiates multiple intracellular signaling cascades that ultimately promote neuronal survival. Key pathways include activation of phosphatidylinositol 3-kinase (PI3K),

Ras, mitogen-activated protein kinases (MAPKs), and phospholipases C (PLCs). Of particular importance is the PI3K-Akt pathway. Akt, a serine-threonine kinase, phosphorylates the pro-apoptotic protein Bad. Phosphorylated Bad is sequestered by 14-3-3 proteins, preventing it from inhibiting anti-apoptotic Bcl-2 family members. This releases Bcl-2 to promote mitochondrial integrity and prevent cytochrome c release, thereby blocking the intrinsic apoptotic pathway and ensuring neuronal survival.

Mechanisms of Synapse Formation

The formation of synapses represents the final critical step in establishing functional neural circuits. Both neuromuscular junctions and central synapses employ sophisticated molecular mechanisms to ensure that synapses form at appropriate locations and acquire proper functional properties.

The Neuromuscular Junction

The neuromuscular junction has served as a premier model system for understanding synapse formation due to its accessibility and relative simplicity. The basal lamina in the synaptic cleft plays an instructive role in dictating both the formation and morphology of the neuromuscular junction.

Acetylcholine receptor aggregation at the neuromuscular junction involves three complementary mechanisms. First, the motor neuron releases agrin into the synaptic cleft. Agrin activates MuSK (muscle-specific tyrosine kinase) on the muscle fiber through the Lrp4 co-receptor. MuSK signaling ultimately recruits rapsyn, a scaffolding protein that organizes and clusters acetylcholine receptors at the synaptic membrane.

Second, the motor neuron releases neuregulin, which activates ErbB2 family receptor tyrosine kinases on the muscle fiber. ErbB signaling leads to upregulation of acetylcholine receptor transcription specifically in nuclei adjacent to the developing neuromuscular junction. Third, signaling through activated acetylcholine receptors leads to calcium influx, which activates kinase cascades that downregulate receptor expression. At the synapse, neuregulin signaling is dominant and overcomes this downregulation. However, in nuclei distant from the synapse, calcium-mediated downregulation predominates. These three mechanisms work in concert to achieve both clustering of existing receptors and selective upregulation of receptor synthesis at the synaptic site while maintaining low receptor density elsewhere on the muscle fiber.

Congenital myasthenia gravis can result from mutations in MuSK, which cause failure of proper neuromuscular junction formation and result in muscle weakness present from birth.

Central Synapse Formation

Central synapses employ bidirectional signaling mechanisms in which both pre- and postsynaptic cells present cell surface molecules that interact to induce synapse formation. Ephrins and Eph receptors, in addition to their role in axon guidance, participate in synapse formation. Neurexins, located on the presynaptic terminal, interact with neuroligins on the postsynaptic membrane. In the mature brain, neuroligin-1 localizes predominantly to excitatory synapses, while neuroligin-2 localizes to inhibitory synapses. This differential localization may contribute to the establishment of appropriate excitatory-inhibitory balance.

Mutations in neuroligin-3 and neuroligin-4 have been identified in patients with autism spectrum disorders, suggesting that proper synapse formation and maintenance is disrupted in these conditions. Mutations in neuroligins have also been associated with Asperger syndrome. Cadherins, cell adhesion molecules that mediate calcium-dependent homophilic binding, also play important roles in synaptic clustering and stabilization.

Astrocytes provide essential support for synapse formation by supplying cholesterol via apolipoprotein E (ApoE). Niemann-Pick type C disease, which results from defects in intracellular cholesterol transport, illustrates the importance of proper cholesterol trafficking for nervous system function.

Synaptic Elimination and Refinement

An important feature of neuromuscular junction development is synaptic elimination, which occurs without neuronal death. Initially, each muscle fiber is innervated by multiple motor axons. Through a competitive process, the strongest synapse is progressively strengthened while weaker synapses are eliminated, ultimately resulting in single innervation of each muscle fiber. The strength of synaptic transmission determines which synapse survives. Stronger synapses are more effective at clustering acetylcholine receptors and also suppress receptor expression at competing synapses, creating a positive feedback loop. This competitive mechanism ensures optimal neuromuscular connectivity and bears conceptual similarity to lateral inhibition mechanisms such as Notch signaling in neural precursor fate determination.

Gliogenesis and Glial Cell Development

Following the initial phase of neurogenesis, neural progenitors switch to producing glial cells. This transition is controlled by specific transcription factors and signaling molecules that regulate the neurogenic-to-gliogenic switch.

The Neurogenesis to Gliogenesis Transition

Astrocytes represent the most numerous type of macroglial cell in the central nervous system. The switch from neurogenesis to gliogenesis involves the upregulation of transcription factors including Olig1/2 and Sox9, along with transcriptional regulators such as SCL. Neuregulin signaling plays a crucial role in this transition by suppressing neuronal differentiation programs while promoting gliogenic programs.

Different progenitor domains exhibit distinct patterns of neuronal-to-glial switching. The pMN domain, which initially produces motor neurons, switches to producing oligodendrocytes.

The p2 domain transitions from generating interneurons to producing astrocytes. In the subventricular zone, the progression moves from GABAergic interneuron production to astrocyte generation and finally to oligodendrocyte production. These domain-specific patterns ensure that appropriate numbers and types of neurons and glia are generated in each region.

Notch Signaling in Cell Fate Determination

Notch signaling plays an essential role in determining whether a progenitor cell becomes a neuron or a glial cell. Initially, all cells in proneural regions express similar levels of both Notch receptors and Delta ligands. During cell division, slight asymmetries in the distribution of signaling molecules to daughter cells are rapidly amplified through Notch-Delta interactions.

When Notch is activated on a cell, it downregulates that cell's expression of Delta ligand. Consequently, a cell expressing high levels of Delta will strongly activate Notch in neighboring cells, which will then downregulate their Delta expression. This reduces the ability of neighboring cells to activate Notch on the primary cell, allowing Delta expression in the primary cell to increase further. This lateral inhibition mechanism rapidly amplifies initial small differences, resulting in a salt-and-pepper pattern in which cells expressing high Delta levels become neurons while cells with low Delta become glia.

Central to this process is neurogenin, a basic helix-loop-helix transcription factor that regulates Delta expression. Only cells expressing neurogenin are competent to undergo this neuronal-glial fate decision, highlighting the importance of transcriptional priming in developmental fate choices.

Glial Differentiation and Cell Number Control

Platelet-derived growth factor (PDGF) maintains glial progenitors in an undifferentiated and proliferative state. It serves as an essential mitogen for glial precursors. In the absence of PDGF, glial progenitors default to oligodendrocyte differentiation. However, if PDGF is absent but ciliary neurotrophic factor (CNTF) is present, glial progenitors differentiate into astrocytes instead. Mature astrocytes regulate the levels of PDGF and potentially CNTF, creating a feedback mechanism that controls the relative numbers of oligodendrocytes and astrocytes produced. This homeostatic mechanism ensures appropriate glial cell populations for nervous system function.

The neuron-to-Schwann cell ratio in the peripheral nervous system is similarly regulated through feedback mechanisms. Ganglionic neurons produce glial growth factor (GGF), a product of the neuregulin gene. GGF inhibits surrounding cells from becoming neurons and instead induces Schwann cell differentiation. Remarkably, the level of neuregulin signaling also determines the amount of myelin produced by each Schwann cell, providing an additional layer of control over peripheral nerve myelination.

Molecular Organization of Myelinated Axons

Myelinated axons exhibit highly organized molecular domains that are essential for saltatory conduction. The node of Ranvier contains high densities of voltage-gated sodium channels along with scaffolding proteins such as neurofascin and dystroglycan. The paranode, flanking each node, contains Caspr and contactin, which mediate adhesion between the axon and myelin loops. The juxtaparanode region contains voltage-gated potassium channels. The internode comprises the myelinated segments between nodes. Proper formation and maintenance of these molecular domains are essential for rapid nerve conduction.

Various diseases affect myelin and glial development. Cerebral palsy can result from malformation of white matter due to impaired glial development. Multiple sclerosis involves immune-mediated destruction of CNS myelin. Krabbe disease results from deficiency of galactosylceramidase, leading to accumulation of toxic metabolites that destroy oligodendrocytes. Charcot-Marie-Tooth disease encompasses a group of inherited neuropathies affecting peripheral nerve myelin. Guillain-Barré syndrome involves acute immune-mediated demyelination of peripheral nerves.

Critical Periods and Neural Plasticity

The concept of critical periods—developmental windows during which neural circuits are particularly malleable and responsive to environmental influences—has profound implications for understanding both normal development and potential therapeutic interventions.

Defining the Critical Period

The critical period represents the time when neural circuitry is maximally plastic and can be shaped by environmental experience. This period typically extends from the time when GABAergic interneurons migrate into the cortex until these inhibitory synapses mature and stabilize. The timing and duration of critical periods varies across different brain regions and functional systems, but the underlying mechanisms appear to be conserved.

Critical period timing is intimately linked to the development of GABAergic inhibition. Processes that delay maturation of GABAergic interneurons and their synapses extend the critical period, while processes that accelerate GABAergic maturation shorten it. This relationship provides potential therapeutic targets for manipulating plasticity.

Manipulating Critical Period Timing

Several experimental approaches can alter critical period timing. Inhibiting GABAergic maturation by depleting GABA through inhibition of glutamic acid decarboxylase (GAD65) extends the critical period. Similarly, eliminating the perineuronal net, an extracellular matrix structure that surrounds mature neurons, by treatment with chondroitinase extends plasticity. Conversely, accelerating GABAergic maturation through administration of benzodiazepines such as valium, which enhance GABAergic signaling, shortens the critical period. Overexpression of brain-derived neurotrophic factor (BDNF) causes premature maturation of GABAergic neurons, resulting in an early onset of the critical period.

During critical periods, competition between different inputs to cortical columns determines which projections are strengthened and which are eliminated. The winning projection solidifies the circuit architecture, a process observed across all aspects of cortical function including sensory processing, motor control, and higher cognitive functions.

Restoring Plasticity in the Adult Brain

Understanding the mechanisms that close critical periods has led to strategies for reopening plasticity in the adult brain. Breaking down perineuronal nets with chondroitinase can restore juvenile levels of plasticity in adult animals. Inhibiting myelination or blocking-related pathways, such as through knockout of the Nogo receptor (NogoR), can also enhance adult plasticity. These findings raise the possibility of therapeutic interventions to promote recovery after brain injury or to facilitate learning in adults.

Functional and Structural Plasticity

Neural plasticity encompasses both functional changes in synaptic strength and structural changes in connectivity. Autism spectrum disorders can result from mutations in genes critical for synapse maintenance, including neuroligin-3 and MeCP2 (methyl-CpG-binding protein 2). These mutations impair the ability to properly maintain and modify synapses in response to experience, potentially underlying the social and cognitive deficits observed in autism.

Neuronal Migration and Migration Disorders

Following their generation in proliferative zones, neurons must migrate to their appropriate positions within the developing brain. Aberrations in this process result in neuronal migration disorders, which represent important causes of epilepsy and developmental delay.

Modes of Neuronal Migration

Neurons employ different migration strategies depending on their location and final destination. Nuclear translocation involves movement of the nucleus within an elongated cell process and is typical of short-distance migrations. Radial migration, the predominant mode for cortical pyramidal neurons, involves migration along radial glial fibers that extend from the ventricular zone to the pial surface. Non-regular migration describes more circuitous routes taken by specific neuronal populations, particularly GABAergic interneurons.

Radial glia arise from neuroepithelial cells and extend elongated processes from the ventricular zone to the pial surface, serving as guide rails for migrating neurons. Pyramidal neurons arise from radial glial cells through asymmetric division and migrate along these glial fibers in an inside-out pattern, with later-born neurons migrating past earlier-born neurons to reach more superficial positions. This results in the characteristic six-layered structure of the neocortex, with layer VI neurons born first and layer II/III neurons born last.

Periventricular Heterotopia

Periventricular heterotopia results from failure of pyramidal neurons to initiate migration away from the ventricular zone. Affected individuals typically have normal intelligence but suffer from medically intractable epilepsy. This condition is caused by mutations in the X-linked gene encoding filamin A, an actin-binding protein essential for initiating neuronal migration. Because filamin A is also required for blood vessel integrity, complete loss of function is embryonic lethal due to hemorrhage. Therefore, this X-linked dominant condition affects primarily females who have random X-inactivation resulting in mosaic expression of normal and mutant filamin A.

Double Cortex Syndrome and Lissencephaly

Double cortex syndrome and lissencephaly represent a spectrum of disorders caused by defects in neuronal migration along radial glial fibers. These conditions result from mutations in DCX (doublecortin), an X-linked gene encoding a microtubule-associated protein essential for neuronal motility. Males with DCX mutations develop severe lissencephaly (smooth brain lacking normal gyral development) and have profound intellectual disability. Females, due to X-inactivation mosaicism, develop a less severe double cortex syndrome characterized by a band of ectopic gray matter between the ventricles and cortex, along with intellectual disability and severe epilepsy beginning in childhood.

Mutations in LIS1, which encodes another microtubule-guidance protein, also cause lissencephaly. Unlike DCX, LIS1 is autosomal, affecting males and females equally.

Inverted Migration and Reelin

In reelin-deficient mice and humans with RELN mutations, cortical layering is inverted with extensive mixing of layers. Reelin, an extracellular matrix protein secreted by Cajal-Retzius cells in the marginal zone, regulates the stopping point of migrating neurons. Without proper reelin signaling, neurons fail to properly position themselves, resulting in disrupted laminar organization.

Walker-Warburg Syndrome

Walker-Warburg syndrome represents an overmigration disorder in which neurons migrate beyond their normal stopping point, sometimes extending through breaks in the pial surface. This condition results from mutations in genes encoding protein O-mannosyltransferases (POMT1, POMT2, and related genes), which are required for glycosylation of dystroglycan. Improperly glycosylated dystroglycan cannot properly organize the pial basement membrane that normally serves as a barrier to migrating neurons. The resulting breaches in this barrier allow neurons to overmigrate, causing severe cortical malformations.

Tangential Migration of GABAergic Interneurons

GABAergic interneurons undergo a distinctly different migration pattern compared to pyramidal neurons. These inhibitory neurons are generated in the medial ganglionic eminence and migrate tangentially (parallel to the cortical surface) to reach the cortex. Mutations in the ARX gene, which encodes a transcription factor essential for GABAergic neuron development, result in a severe deficit of cortical inhibitory neurons. Affected individuals experience intense epilepsy due to lack of cortical inhibition. ARX mutations represent an X-linked recessive disorder typically affecting only males.

Once GABAergic interneurons reach the cortex, neuregulin signaling through ErbB4 receptors guides their migration within cortical layers to reach appropriate positions. This ensures proper distribution of inhibitory neurons throughout the cortex, which is essential for balanced excitatory-inhibitory neurotransmission.

Mechanisms Limiting and Promoting Spinal Cord Regeneration

Unlike peripheral nerves, which retain substantial regenerative capacity, central nervous system axons exhibit very limited regrowth after injury. Understanding the factors that limit CNS regeneration represents an active area of research with important therapeutic implications for spinal cord injury.

Intrinsic Limiting Factors

Mature CNS neurons have limited intrinsic capacity for axonal regrowth, which contrasts with the robust growth potential of developing neurons. This age-dependent decline in regenerative capacity results from expression of specific cell cycle regulatory genes that control axonal growth programs. The retinoblastoma protein (pRB), p53, PTEN, and TSC1 all suppress axonal growth in mature neurons.

Deletion of PTEN (phosphatase and tensin homolog) has emerged as a particularly promising approach for promoting axonal regeneration. PTEN inhibits the PI3K/Akt signaling pathway, which in turn activates mTOR (mammalian target of rapamycin). The mTOR pathway is critical for axonal growth, and its activity declines as neurons mature. Experimental deletion of PTEN in mature neurons reactivates the PI3K/Akt/mTOR pathway and promotes robust axonal regrowth after injury.

Extrinsic Inhibitory Factors

In addition to intrinsic limitations, the environment of the injured CNS actively inhibits axonal regeneration. Myelin debris from injured oligodendrocytes and Schwann cells contains multiple inhibitory molecules that block growth cone formation and neurite outgrowth. Three major myelin-associated inhibitors have been identified: Nogo-A, myelin-associated glycoprotein (MAG), and oligodendrocyte-myelin glycoprotein (OMgp).

All three of these inhibitors bind to the Nogo receptor (NogoR) and its co-receptor PirB (paired immunoglobulin-like receptor B). Blocking NogoR function, either through antibody neutralization (using the IN-1 antibody) or genetic deletion, allows increased neurite growth after injury. This has led to ongoing clinical trials evaluating anti-Nogo antibodies for spinal cord injury treatment.

Promoting Regeneration

Several approaches beyond blocking inhibitory signals can promote axonal regeneration. Local application of neurotrophic factors, particularly neurotrophin-3, can stimulate neurite growth by activating Trk receptor signaling and downstream growth-promoting pathways. Enzymatic digestion of the extracellular matrix, especially chondroitin sulfate proteoglycans that accumulate in the glial scar, can also facilitate regrowth. Interestingly, these manipulations are conceptually similar to strategies for reopening critical periods—both involve degrading inhibitory extracellular matrix components and reactivating developmental growth programs.

The challenge of spinal cord regeneration illustrates how understanding developmental mechanisms can inform therapeutic strategies. By identifying the molecular brakes that normally prevent regeneration and finding ways to release them, researchers are working toward treatments that could restore function after devastating CNS injuries.

Conclusion

Neurodevelopment encompasses an extraordinarily complex series of cellular and molecular events that must be precisely coordinated to generate a functional nervous system. From the initial formation of the neural tube through the final refinement of synaptic connections, each stage depends on specific signaling pathways, transcription factors, and cell-cell interactions. Clinical observations of developmental disorders have proven invaluable in identifying key molecules and mechanisms, while basic research continues to reveal new layers of complexity in neural development. Understanding these processes provides essential foundation for comprehending not only developmental neuropathology but also the potential for regeneration and plasticity in the mature nervous system. As research progresses, insights from developmental neurobiology increasingly inform therapeutic strategies for neurological injury and disease, highlighting the enduring clinical relevance of this fundamental field.

Index

A
Abducens nerve, 42
Abnormal movements, types of, 136
Acalculia, 148, 159
Accessory nerve, 49
Achromatopsia, 162
Acquired hydrocephalus, 197
Addiction, 171, 172, 180
Afferent fibers, 83
  climbing fibers, 84
  modulatory afferent systems, 85–86
  mossy fibers, 84
  parallel fibers, 85
Afferent pupillary defect, 67
Agranular cortex, 142
Agraphia, 148, 158, 159
Alexia without agraphia, 186
Alzheimer's disease, 173–176, 187
  APP processing, 174–175
  excitotoxicity, 175–176
  genetics, 176
  neuropathological hallmarks, 174
  therapeutic strategies, 176
Amygdala, 169
Amygdalar pathways, 170
Amyloid precursor protein (APP) processing, 174–175
Amyotrophic lateral sclerosis (ALS), 19, 187
Anosmia, 65
Ansa lenticularis, 132
Anterior cerebral artery (ACA), 206, 209, 210, 226, 227
Anterior choroidal artery, 205, 228
Anterior cingulate cortex (ACC), 156
Anterior cingulotomy, 156, 168
Anterior circulation strokes, 226–227
Anterior communicating artery, 209
Anterior cord syndrome, 18
Anterior corticospinal tract, 13
Anterior inferior cerebellar artery (AICA), 207, 212
Anterior intralaminar group, 111
Anterior spinal artery, 207, 223–225
Anteromedial hypothalamus activation, 115
Anxiety disorders, 173
Aphasias, 185–187
Apolipoprotein E (APOE) polymorphisms, 176
Aqueduct of Sylvius, 192
Archicerebellar syndrome, 87
Arnold-Chiari malformation, 99
Arterial supply, 14, 223–224

V. Yanamadala, *Essential Neuroanatomy*,
https://doi.org/10.1007/978-3-032-26877-8

Arteria radicularis magna, 224
Artery of Adamkiewicz, 224
Ascending reticular activating system (ARAS), 36
Ascending (sensory) tracts, 12
Association cortices, 147, 148
Association fibers, 181
Astrocytes, 249
Asynergia, 90
Ataxia, 97
Auditory and language areas, 152
Auditory hallucinations, 167
Auditory processing, 164
Auriculotemporal nerve, 76
Autism spectrum disorder, 180
Autonomic innervation, 222
Autonomic nervous system, 10
Autonomic regulation, 177, 180
Axonal guidance mechanisms, 241
  dendrites, 244
  ephrins, 243
  morphogen signaling, 244–245
  netrins, 241
  Robo receptors, 242
  semaphorins, 242
  slits, 242
  switching guidance responses, 243, 244
  topographic mapping, 243

B

Balance, 95
Balint syndrome, 159
Basal ganglia
  abnormal movements, types of, 136
  arterial supply, 132–133
  basal ganglia, 128–129
  caudate nucleus, 124
  clinical disorders
    carbon monoxide toxicity, 136
    choreoathetosis, 136
    dentatorubropallidoluysian atrophy, 136
    dystonia, 135
    hemiballismus, 135
    Huntington's disease, 134
    methanol toxicity, 136
    Parkinson's disease, 133–134
    tardive dyskinesia, 135
    Tourette syndrome, 135, 136
  functional anatomy and neural pathways, 126–128
  functional circuitry, 131
  globus pallidus, 125
  major fiber pathways, 131–132
  motor control, 128–129
  neuroanatomical organization, 129, 130
  output targets, 132
  putamen, 124
  STN, 125
  substantia nigra, 125
Basal vein of Rosenthal, 217
Basket cells, 82, 83
Behavioral and personality changes, 157
Bell-Magendie law, 10
Bergmann cells, 82, 83
Bergmann gliosis, 83
Bilateral trochlear nerve palsy, 72
Bipolar disorder, 173
Blood-brain barrier (BBB), 218
  circumventricular organs, 220
  clinical significance, 220
  selective permeability, 219
  structural basis, 218, 219
Blood pressure maintenance, 27
Bone morphogenetic proteins (BMPs), 240, 244
Brain death, 58
Brain-derived neurotrophic factor (BDNF), 245, 246, 253
Brainstem
  autonomic and vital functions, 58

cholinergic system, 52, 53
consciousness and arousal, 58
cranial nerve functions, 59
dopaminergic systems, 50–51
histaminergic system, 53
major brainstem tracts, 53–56
central tegmental tract, 54
lateral lemniscus, 55
medial forebrain bundle, 56
medial lemniscus, 55
MLF, 53–54
posterior (dorsal) longitudinal fasciculus, 54
trigeminothalamic tracts, 55
medulla oblongata, 42
anatomical structures, 47–48
cerebellar peduncles, 48
cranial nerves, 49–50
critical functional centers, 46
vascular supply, 57
midbrain, 31
anatomical organization, 32–36
cranial nerves, 36
vascular supply, 56
motor control and coordination, 58
noradrenergic system, 51
pons, 37
anatomical features, 38–41
cranial nerves, 41–42
vascular supply, 56–57
sensory processing and relay, 58
serotonergic system, 52–53
vascular supply, 57
Broca's aphasia, 185
Broca's area, 148
Brown-Séquard syndrome, 17
Buccal nerve, 76

C

Carbon monoxide toxicity, 136
Cardiovascular centers, 46
Cardiovascular regulation, 27
Carrier-mediated transport, 219
Cauda equina syndrome, 18, 226
Caudate nucleus, 124
Cavernous sinuses, 215
Central canal, 6, 192
Central (transtentorial) herniation, 230
Central cord syndrome, 17–18
Central nervous system (CNS), 1, 27
anterior cerebral artery territory, 210
BBB, 218
circumventricular organs, 220
clinical significance, 220
selective permeability, 219
structural basis, 218, 219
cerebellar artery territories, 211–212
cerebral autoregulation, 220–222
cerebral herniation, 228–231
cerebral venous drainage, 212–218
circle of Willis, 208–209
collateral circulation, 208–209
hemodynamics, 220–222
internal carotid arteries, 204, 206
intracranial hemorrhage, 231–234
middle cerebral artery territory, 210–211
posterior cerebral artery, 211
stroke syndromes, 226
anterior circulation, 226–227
deep structure, 228
posterior circulation, 227
vertebrobasilar system, 206–208
Central tegmental tract, 54
Central vision, 67
Centromedian nucleus, 111

Cerebellar artery territories, 211–212
Cerebellar connections, 38–39
Cerebellar cortex, 81
  afferent fibers
    climbing fibers, 84
    modulatory afferent systems, 85–86
    mossy fibers, 84
    parallel fibers, 85
  cortical cell types, 82–83
  cortical layers, 81–82
Cerebellar hypoplasia, 100
Cerebellar learning mechanisms, 96
Cerebellar peduncles, 48
Cerebellum
  anatomical organization, 79–80
  cerebellar cortex, 81
    afferent fibers, 83–86
    cortical cell types, 82–83
    cortical layers, 81–82
  Chiari malformations, 98–100
  deep cerebellar nuclei
    dentate nucleus, 91–92
    efferent pathways, 93–95
    fastigial nucleus, 92–93
    interposed nuclei, 92
    nuclear organization, 91
  functional divisions
    cerebrocerebellum, 88–91
    spinocerebellum, 87–88
    vestibulocerebellum, 86–87
  functions, 96
  neoplastic conditions, 98
  signs and symptoms, 97–98
Cerebral autoregulation, 220–222
Cerebral blood flow, 221
Cerebral cortex
  Alzheimer's disease
    APP processing, 174–175
    excitotoxicity, 175–176
    genetics, 176
    neuropathological hallmarks, 174
    therapeutic strategies, 176
  association cortices, 147, 148
  Brodmann's cytoarchitectonic map and functional correlates, 150
    auditory and language areas, 152
    left hemisphere dominance, 153
    parietal association areas, 153
    prefrontal and executive areas, 152
    right hemisphere dominance, 153
    somatosensory association areas, 152
    visual and visuospatial areas, 151
  clinical syndromes, 185–187
  cortical communications
    intracortical communications, 180–181
    subcortical communications, 181–182
  cortical plasticity and reorganization, 154
  frontal lobe
    anatomical boundaries and subdivisions, 155–156
    clinical syndromes, 156–157
    major white matter connections, 156
  functional organization, 142–149
  general structure, 140–142
  insula, 177
    anatomical organization, 177
    autonomic regulation, 178–179
    bodily awareness, 178

clinical disorders, 179
decision-making and risk processing, 179
emotional processing and regulation, 178
empathy, 178
interoception, 178
social cognition, 178
language centers, 148, 149
limbic system (*see* Limbic system)
motor cortices, 145, 146
occipital lobe
anatomical organization, 160
clinical syndromes, 161–163
hierarchical visual processing, 161
retinotopic organization, 160
visual field representation, 160
parietal lobe, 157
anatomical subdivisions, 158
clinical syndromes, 159
functional specializations, 158
primary sensory cortices
primary auditory cortex, 144
primary gustatory cortex, 145
primary olfactory cortex, 145
primary somatosensory cortex, 143
primary visual cortex, 143, 144
stroke syndromes, 182–184
temporal lobe
additional temporal lobe structures, 164
clinical syndromes, 166–167
functional domains, 164–165
gross anatomical organization, 163–164
vascular supply, 182–184
Cerebral hemispheres, 140, 153, 182
Cerebral herniation, 228–231
Cerebral palsy, 251
Cerebral peduncles, 34
Cerebral venous drainage, 212–218
Cerebrocerebellum, 88–91
Cerebrospinal fluid (CSF), 1, 6, 15, 193–194
Charcot-Marie-Tooth disease, 251
Chemoaffinity hypothesis, 243
Chiari type 0 malformation, 100
Chiari type I malformation, 98–99
Chiari type II malformation, 99
Chiari type III malformation, 100
Chiari type IV malformation, 100
Cholinergic fibers, 86
Cholinergic system, 52, 53
Choreoathetosis, 136
Chronic rhinosinusitis, 65
Ciliary muscle, 69
Ciliary neurotrophic factor (CNTF), 251
Cingulate (subfalcine) herniation, 230
Cingulate gyrus, 167
Circle of Willis, 203, 205, 208–209
Circumventricular organs, 116, 220
Clarke's nucleus, 11
Climbing fibers, 84
Cognitive and emotional processing, 96
Collateral circulation, 208–209
Commissural fibers, 181
Communicating hydrocephalus, 195
Complex visual phenomena, 163
Conduction aphasia, 185
Congenital anosmia, in Kallmann syndrome, 65
Congenital hydrocephalus, 196
Congenital myasthenia gravis, 248
Consolidation, 165
Conus medullaris syndrome, 18

Corneal reflex tests, 77
Corpus callosotomy, 185
Cortical cell types, 82–83
Cortical communications
  intracortical communications, 180–181
  subcortical communications, 181–182
Cortical layers, 81–82
Cortical plasticity, 154
Cortical reorganization, 154
Corticopontocerebellar pathway, 39
Corticostriatal fibers, 182
Corticostriatal projections, 156
Cranial nerves
  functions, 59
  oculomotor nerve
    clinical relevance, 68–70
    course and distribution, 68
    functional classification, 68
    nuclear organization, 68
    parasympathetic pathway, 69
  olfactory nerve, 64–65
  optic nerve
    central vision, 67
    clinical relevance, 67
    course of, 66
    decussation, 66
    embryological significance, 65
    functional classification, 65
    optic chiasm, 66
    optic tracts, 67
    retinal organization, 66
  trigeminal nerve
    clinical relevance, 72–78
    functional classification, 72
    mandibular division, 75
    maxillary division, 74
    nuclear organization, 73
    ophthalmic division, 74
    overview, 72
  trochlear nerve
    clinical relevance, 71, 72
    course and distribution, 71
    functional classification, 70
    nuclear origin and unique anatomical features, 70
    superior oblique muscle, 71
Critical period, 252
Cyclic AMP (cAMP), 243
Cyclic GMP (cGMP), 243, 244

D

Decompensated congenital trochlear palsy, 72
Decomposition of movements, 90
Deep cerebellar nuclei
  dentate nucleus, 91–92
  efferent pathways, 93–95
  fastigial nucleus, 92–93
  interposed nuclei, 92
  nuclear organization, 91
Deep cerebral venous drainage, 216–218
Deep intracerebral hemorrhage, 234
Deep structure strokes, 228
Degenerative and demyelinating disorders, 19–20
Dentate nucleus efferents, 93
Dentatorubropallidoluysian atrophy (DRPLA), 136
Descending (motor) tracts, 13
Diencephalon
  epithalamus
    habenular complex, 116–117
    overview and components, 116
    pineal gland, 117–118
  hypothalamus
    anterior-posterior organization, 112–113
    circumventricular organs, 116
    major afferent pathways, 114
    major efferent pathways, 115
    medial-lateral organization, 113–114

overview and functional significance, 112
physiological and behavioral responses, 115
structural and functional divisions, 103
subthalamus, 118, 119
thalamus
anterior group, 107
anterior intralaminar group, 111
dorsomedial nucleus, 107–108
functional classification, 107
lateral dorsal nucleus, 108
lateral geniculate nucleus, 110
lateral posterior nucleus, 108
medial geniculate nucleus, 111
midline nuclei, 108
poterior intralaminar group, 111
pulvinar, 108
structural organization, 105
thalamic reticular nucleus, 111
ventral anterior nucleus, 109
ventral lateral nucleus, 109
ventral posterolateral nucleus, 109
ventral posteromedial nucleus, 109–110
vascular supply, 119–120
Diffuse projection systems, 182
Disconnection syndromes, 185
Dopamine, 51
Dopaminergic fibers, 85–86
Dopaminergic modulation of movement, 128
Dopaminergic systems, 50–51
Dorsal column-medial lemniscal pathway, 9
Dorsal column nuclei, 48
Dorsal root ganglia, 11
Dorsal-ventral patterning, 241
Dorsolateral prefrontal cortex (DLPFC), 147, 155
Dorsomedial nucleus functions, 107
Double cortex syndrome, 255
Down syndrome cell adhesion molecule (DSCAM), 244
Downward cerebellar (tonsillar) herniation, 231
Dual-pathway system, 170
Dural venous sinuses, 212–215
Dysdiadochokinesia, 90
Dysmetria, 90, 97
Dystonia, 135

E

Edinger-Westphal nucleus, 68–70
Efflux transporters, 219
Emboliform, 92
Emotional and psychiatric disorders, 179
Emotional dysregulation, 167
Emotional processing, 165
Endoscopic third ventriculostomy (ETV), 200
Entorhinal cortex, 64
EphA2 receptors, 244
Eph receptors, 243, 248
Epithalamus
habenular complex, 116–117
overview and components, 116
pineal gland, 117–118
Executive dysfunction, 157
Extensive reciprocal connections, 156
Extradural (epidural) hemorrhage, 231
Extrapyramidal tracts, 13
Extrinsic inhibitory factors, 257

F

Facial nerve, 42
Facilitation of movement, 126

Fasciculus retroflexus, 117
Fastigial nucleus, 87, 88, 92, 94
Finger agnosia, 148, 159
Fornix, 114, 115, 170
Fourth ventricle, 192
Frontal eye fields, 146, 157
Frontal lobe, 140
  anatomical boundaries and subdivisions, 155–156
  clinical syndromes, 156–157
  major white matter connections, 156
Frontal nerve, 74
Frontotemporal dementia, 186
Functional and structural plasticity, 253
Functional circuitry, 131

G
GABAergic interneurons, 256
Generalized anxiety disorder, 173, 179
Gerstmann syndrome, 148, 159
Geschwind's disconnection syndromes, 186
Glaucoma, 68
Glial cell development, 249–252
Glial growth factor (GGF), 251
Gliogenesis, 249–252
Globose, 92
Globus pallidus, 125
Glomeruli, 64
Glossopharyngeal nerve, 49
Glutamate excitotoxicity, 175
Glutamate transporters, 175
Golgi cells, 82–85
Granular cortex, 142
Granular layer, 82
Granule cells, 82
Gray matter of the brain, *see* Cerebral cortex
Great cerebral vein of Galen, 217
Guillain-Barré syndrome, 252
Guillain-Mollaret triangle, *see* Mollaret's triangle

H
Habenulointerpeduncular tract, 117
Hemiballismus, 119, 121, 135
Hemisection, 17
Hemodynamics, 220–222
Herniated intervertebral disc, 23
Heterotypic cortex, 142
Hierarchical visual processing, 161
Hippocampus, 168, 169
Histaminergic system, 53
Homotypic cortex, 142
Horizontal gaze palsy with progressive scoliosis (HGPPS), 244
Huntington's disease, 134
Hydrocephalus
  classification
    acquired, 197
    communicating, 195
    congenital, 196
    non-communicating, 195
    normal pressure, 196
  clinical manifestations, 197–199
  diagnosis, 199
  long-term management, 201
  pathophysiology, 197
  prognosis, 201
  treatment, 200
Hypoglossal nerve, 49
Hypophyseotropic tract, 115
Hyporeflexia, 90
Hyposmia, 65
Hypothalamic-pituitary-adrenal (HPA) axis, 172
Hypothalamohypophyseal tract, 115
Hypothalamomedullary tract, 115
Hypothalamospinal tract, 115
Hypothalamus, 171
  anterior-posterior organization, 112–113

circumventricular organs, 116
major afferent pathways, 114
major efferent pathways, 115
medial-lateral organization, 113–114
overview and functional significance, 112
physiological and behavioral responses, 115
Hypotonia, 90

I
Infectious disorders, 21–22
Inferior alveolar nerve, 76
Inferior colliculi, 32
Inferior mammillary peduncle, 114
Inferior olivary nuclear complex, 47–48
Inferior sagittal sinus, 213
Inflammatory disorders, 20
Infraorbital nerve, 75
Inhibition of movement, 128
Insula, 177
anatomical organization, 177
autonomic regulation, 178–179
bodily awareness, 178
clinical disorders, 179
decision-making and risk processing, 179
emotional processing and regulation, 178
empathy, 178
interoception, 178
social cognition, 178
Intention tremor, 90, 97
Internal carotid arteries (ICA), 204–206, 209
Internal cerebral veins, 216
Interpeduncular nucleus, 36
Interposed nuclei efferents, 93
Interstitial nucleus of Cajal (INC), 35
Intracranial hemorrhage, 231–234
Intraventricular hemorrhage, 234
Intrinsic vascular supply, 224
Inverted migration, 255
Irritable bowel syndrome, 180

K
Korsakoff syndrome, 173
Krabbe disease, 251

L
Lacrimal nerve, 74
Language centers, 148, 149
Language comprehension, 164–165
Language disorders, 157
Lateral corticospinal tract, 13
Lateral dorsal nucleus, 108, 111
Lateral geniculate nucleus (LGN), 67, 110
Lateral habenular nucleus, 117
Lateral lemniscus, 55
Lateral posterior nucleus, 108
Lateral temporal cortex, 148
Lateral ventricles, 190–191
Left hemisphere dominance, 153
Left insular cortex, 114
Left-right disorientation, 148, 159
Lenticular fasciculus, 132
Lenticular nucleus, 130
Lenticulostriate artery occlusion, 228
Lesions of Meyer's loop, 67
Limbic basal ganglia, 171
Limbic circuit (anterior cingulate), 131
Limbic system
clinical disorders, 173
functional roles, 172–173
principal components
amygdala, 169
amygdalar pathways, 170
cingulate gyrus, 167
fornix, 170
hippocampus, 168, 169

Limbic system (*cont.*)
hypothalamus, 171
limbic basal ganglia, 171
mammillary bodies, 171
parahippocampal gyrus, 168
rapid emotional response system, 170
septal nuclei, 171
Lingual nerve, 76
Lissencephaly, 255
Lobar intracerebral hemorrhage, 233
Locus coeruleus (LC), 41
Long circumferential penetrators, 57

M
Main sensory nucleus, 73
Major brainstem tracts, 53–56
central tegmental tract, 54
lateral lemniscus, 55
medial forebrain bundle, 56
medial lemniscus, 55
MLF, 53–54
posterior (dorsal) longitudinal fasciculus, 54
trigeminothalamic tracts, 55
Major depressive disorder, 173
Major fiber pathways, 131–132
Major spinal nerve plexuses, 8
Mammillary bodies, 171
Marcus Gunn pupil, 67
Matrix, 129
Medial forebrain bundle, 56, 114, 115
Medial geniculate nucleus (MGN), 111
Medial habenular nucleus, 117
Medial lemniscus, 55
Medial longitudinal fasciculus (MLF), 42, 53–54
Median eminence, 51
Medulla oblongata, 28, 42
anatomical structures, 47–48
cerebellar peduncles, 48
cranial nerves, 49–50
critical functional centers, 46
vascular supply, 57
Medullary respiratory centers, 47
Medulloblastoma, 98
Melatonin synthesis, 117, 118
Memory disorders, 173
Memory formation, 165
Meningeal branch (nervus spinosus), 75, 76
Meningeal layers, 15
Mesencephalic nucleus, 73
Mesencephalon, *see* Midbrain
Metabotropic glutamate receptors (mGluRs), 175
Metastatic spinal tumors, 24–25
Metencephalon, *see* Pons
Methanol toxicity, 136
Midbrain (mesencephalon), 27, 31–37
anatomical organization
cerebral peduncles, 34, 35
nuclei, 35, 36
tectum, 32–33
tegmentum, 33, 34
cranial nerves, 36
vascular supply, 56
Middle cerebral artery (MCA), 182, 205, 206, 210, 211, 226, 227
Midline nuclei, 108
Mitogen-activated protein kinases (MAPKs), 247
Modulatory afferent systems, 85–86
Molecular layer, 81–82
Mollaret's triangle, 94
Mood disorders, 173
Morphogen signaling, 245
Mossy fibers, 84
Motion blindness, 162
Motor branches, 75
Motor circuit (primary motor cortex), 131
Motor coordination, 95
Motor cortices, 145, 146
Motor deficits, 156–157
Motor function, 8–9

Motor initiation, 129
Motor learning, 95–96, 129
Motor nucleus, 73
Motor pathways, 3
Motor suppression, 129
Motor system projections, 182
Movement coordination, 129
Multiple sclerosis (MS), 19, 20
Myelencephalon, *see* Medulla oblongata
Myelinated axons, 251

N

Nasal polyps, 65
Nasociliary nerve, 74
Neocerebellar syndrome, 90–91
Neocerebellum, *see* Cerebrocerebellum
Neoplastic disorders, 24–25
Nerve growth factor (NGF), 245, 246
Neural activity, 222
Neural crest, 239–241
Neural plasticity, 253
Neural tube closure, 238
Neural tube defects, 238, 239
Neuregulin signaling, 249
Neurodegenerative patterns, 186–187
Neurodevelopment
  axonal guidance mechanisms, 241
    dendrites, 244
    ephrins, 243
    netrins, 241
    Robo receptors, 242
    semaphorins, 242
    slits, 242
    switching guidance responses, 243, 244
    topographic mapping, 243
  CNS regeneration, 257, 258
  critical period, 252
  glial cell development, 249–252
  gliogenesis, 249–252
  migration disorders
    double cortex syndrome, 255
    GABAergic interneurons, 256
    inverted migration, 255
    lissencephaly, 255
    modes of, 254
    periventricular heterotopia, 254
    reelin, 255
    Walker-Warburg syndrome, 256
  morphogen signaling, 244–245
  neural progenitor populations, 239–241
  neural tube closure, 238
  neural tube defects, 238, 239
  neuronal survival, 245, 246
  neurotrophin signaling, 245–247
  plasticity, 253
  primary neurulation, 237
  regional specification, 239–241
  secondary neurulation, 238
  synapse formation, mechanisms of, 247
    central synapse formation, 248
    neuromuscular junction, 247
    synaptic elimination and refinement, 249
Neuromuscular junction, 247–249
Neuromyelitis optica spectrum disorder (NMOSD), 20
Neuronal migration and migration disorders
  double cortex syndrome, 255
  GABAergic interneurons, 256
  inverted migration, 255
  lissencephaly, 255
  modes of, 254
  periventricular heterotopia, 254
  reelin, 255
  Walker-Warburg syndrome, 256
Neuronal survival, 245, 246
Neuronal-to-glial switching, 249

Neurotrophin-receptor pairs, 246
Neurotrophin signaling, 245–247
Neurotrophin-3 (NT3), 245, 246
Node of Ranvier, 251
Non-communicating hydrocephalus, 195
Non-regular migration, 254
Noradrenergic fibers, 85
Noradrenergic system, 51
Normal pressure hydrocephalus (NPH), 196
Notch signaling, 249, 250
Nuclear translocation, 254
Nucleus accumbens, 130
Nucleus of Darkschewitsch, 36
Nystagmus, 91, 97–98

O

Obstructive hydrocephalus, 195, 200
Occipital lobe, 140
  anatomical organization, 160
  clinical syndromes, 161–163
  hierarchical visual processing, 161
  retinotopic organization, 160
  visual field representation, 160
Oculomotor apraxia, 159
Oculomotor nerve, 37
  clinical relevance, 68–70
  course and distribution, 68
  functional classification, 68
  nuclear organization, 68
  parasympathetic pathway, 69
Olfactory fila, 64, 65
Olfactory groove meningiomas, 65
Olfactory nerve, 64–65
Olfactory receptor neurons, 64
Onuf's nucleus, 11
Ophthalmic artery, 205
Ophthalmic division, 74
Optic ataxia, 159
Optic chiasm, 66, 67
Optic nerve
  central vision, 67
  clinical relevance, 67
  course of, 66
  decussation, 66
  embryological significance, 65
  functional classification, 65
  optic chiasm, 66
  optic tracts, 67
  retinal organization, 66
Optic neuritis, 67
Optic tracts, 67
Orbitofrontal cortex (OFC), 147, 155

P

p2 domain, 250
PaCO2, 221
Pain disorders, 179
Pallidohypothalamic fibers, 114
Pallidum, *see* Globus pallidus
Panic disorder, 173
PaO2, 222
Papilledema, 67
Parabigeminal nucleus, 36
Parafascicular nucleus, 111
Parahippocampal gyrus, 164, 168
Parallel fibers, 85
Paramedian perforators, 57
Parietal association areas, 153
Parietal lobe, 140, 157–159
Parkinson's disease, 133–134
Parks-Bielschowsky three-step test, 72
Parosmia, 65
Pars compacta, 126
Pars magnocellularis, 107, 109
Pars multiformis (paralaminaris), 108
Pars parvocellularis, 108–110
Pars principalis, 109
Pars reticulata, 126
PAX genes, 241
Pedunculopontine nucleus (PPN), 36
Pendular reflexes, 90
Periaqueductal gray (PAG), 34
Periventricular heterotopia, 254

Phantosmia, 65
Phosphatidylinositol 3-kinase (PI3K), 246, 247, 257
Phospholipases C (PLCs), 247
Phrenic nucleus, 11
PI3K-Akt pathway, 247
Pick's disease, 186
Pilocytic astrocytoma, 98
Pineal gland, 117–118
Platelet-derived growth factor (PDGF), 250, 251
pMN domain, 249
Polymodal association cortex, 170
Pons, 27, 37
  anatomical features, 38–41
  cranial nerves, 41–42
  vascular supply, 56–57
Pontine arteries, 207
Pontine nuclei, 38
Pontine respiratory centers, 40
Pontine respiratory group, 40
Posterior cerebral artery (PCA), 119, 205, 208, 209, 211, 227
Posterior choroidal artery occlusion, 228
Posterior circulation strokes, 227
Posterior communicating artery, 119, 205, 209
Posterior cord syndrome, 18
Posterior inferior cerebellar artery (PICA), 46, 57, 207, 212, 227
Posterior longitudinal fasciculus, 54
Posterior parietal cortex, 147, 158
Posterior spinal artery, 223, 225
Posterior vein of the corpus callosum, 217
Posterolateral hypothalamus activation, 115
Post-traumatic stress disorder (PTSD), 173, 179
Postural control, 129
Posture, 95
Poterior intralaminar group, 111
Pott's disease, 22
Prefrontal and executive areas, 152
Prefrontal circuit, 131
Prefrontal cortex, 147, 150, 155, 177
Premotor cortex, 146, 155
Presenilin 1 (PSEN1), 176
Presenilin 2 (PSEN2), 176
Primary auditory cortex, 144
Primary gustatory cortex, 145
Primary intramedullary tumors, 24
Primary motor cortex, 145, 155
Primary neurulation, 237
Primary olfactory cortex, 145
Primary sensory cortices, 143–145
Primary somatosensory cortex, 143
Primary visual cortex, 143, 144
Prolactin-inhibiting hormone, 51
Pterygopalatine nerves, 75
Pupil-involving palsies, 70
Pupil-sparing palsies, 70
Purkinje cells, 82–87, 91, 96
Putamen, 124
Pyramids, 47

R

Radial migration, 254
Raphe nuclei, 52
Rapid emotional response system, 170
Ras, 247
Rebound phenomenon, 90
Receptor-mediated transcytosis, 219
Recurrent artery of Heubner occlusion, 228
Red nucleus, 33, 119
Reelin, 255
Reflex circuits, 10
Retinohypothalamic tract, 114
Right hemisphere dominance, 153
Right insular cortex, 114
Rostral interstitial nucleus of the medial longitudinal fasciculus (riMLF), 35

S
Scanning speech, 91
Schizophrenia, 167, 180
Schwann cell differentiation, 251
Secondary neurulation, 238
Segmental and radicular arteries, 223
Semaphorin 3A, 242, 244
Sensory branches, 76
Sensory function, 9
Sensory pathways, 3
Septal nuclei, 171
Septal veins, 217
Serotonergic fibers, 86
Serotonergic system, 52–53
Short circumferential penetrators, 57
Short-distance migrations, 254
Sigmoid sinuses, 215
Signaling endosome model, 246
Somatosensory association areas, 152
Sonic Hedgehog (SHH) signaling, 245
Speech production centers, 156
Sphincter pupillae muscle, 69
Spinal accessory nucleus, 11
Spinal cord
    arterial supply, 223–224
    ascending tracts, 12
    clinical syndromes, 225–226
    degenerative and demyelinating disorders, 19–20
    descending tracts, 13
    embryological development, 16
    functional organization
        autonomic function, 10
        and clinical significance, 11
        essential anatomical principles, 10–11
        motor function, 8–9
        reflex circuits, 10
        sensory function, 9
    gross anatomy, 2–4
    infectious disorders, 21–22
    inflammatory disorders, 20
    internal anatomy
        central canal, 6
        gray matter organization, 4–5
        white matter organization, 5–6
    intrinsic vascular supply, 224
    neoplastic disorders, 24–25
    organization, 239–240
    protective structures, 15
    regeneration
        challenges, 258
        extrinsic inhibitory factors, 257
        intrinsic limiting factors, 257
        promoting, 258
    spinal nerves and root organization, 7–8
    structural and compressive disorders, 22–23
    traumatic spinal cord injury
        anterior cord syndrome, 18
        Brown-Séquard Syndrome, 17
        central cord syndrome, 17–18
        complete transection, 17
        conus medullaris vs. cauda equina syndrome, 18
        posterior cord syndrome, 18
    vascular disorders, 21
    vascular supply, 13, 14
    venous drainage, 225
Spinal cord disorders, 1
Spinal cord infarction, 21
Spinal cord ischemia, 21
Spinal epidural abscess, 21–22
Spinal hemorrhage, 21
Spinal muscular atrophy (SMA), 19–20
Spinal stenosis, 22–23
Spinal trigeminal nucleus, 73
Spinobulbocerebellum, *see* Spinocerebellum
Spinocerebellar tracts, 3, 9, 12
Spinocerebellum, 87–88
Spinothalamic tract, 9, 12

Stellate cells, 81, 83
Stereotactic radiofrequency ablation, 156
Straight sinus, 213
Stria medullaris, 117
Striatal architecture, 129
Stria terminalis, 114, 170
Striosomes, 129
Stroke syndromes
  anterior circulation, 226–227
  deep structure, 228
  posterior circulation, 227
Structural and compressive disorders, 22–23
Subarachnoid hemorrhage, 233
Subcortical communications, 181–182
Subcortical projection systems, 181
Subdural hemorrhage, 233
Substantia nigra, 34, 50, 119, 125
Subthalamic fasciculus, 131
Subthalamus, 118, 119
Superior cerebellar artery (SCA), 207, 208, 212
Superior cerebellar veins, 218
Superior colliculi, 32
Superior oblique muscle, 71
Superior sagittal sinus, 212
Supplementary motor area (SMA), 146
Sydenham's chorea, 136
Synapse formation, 247
  central synapse formation, 248
  neuromuscular junction, 247
  synaptic elimination and refinement, 249
Syringomyelia, 23

T

Tardive dyskinesia, 135
Tectum, 32
Telephone cord, 1
Temporal lobe, 140
  clinical syndromes, 166–167
  epilepsy, 166
  functional domains, 164–165
  gross anatomical organization, 163–164
  structures, 164
Thalamic fasciculus, 132
Thalamic reticular nucleus, 111
Thalamocortical and corticothalamic fibers, 181
Thalamogeniculate arteries, 119, 228
Thalamohypothalamic fibers, 114
Thalamoperforating artery occlusion, 228
Thalamostriate (terminal) vein, 217
Thalamus
  anterior group, 107
  anterior intralaminar group, 111
  dorsomedial nucleus, 107–108
  functional classification, 107
  lateral dorsal nucleus, 108
  lateral geniculate nucleus, 110
  lateral posterior nucleus, 108
  medial geniculate nucleus, 111
  midline nuclei, 108
  poterior intralaminar group, 111
  pulvinar, 108
  structural organization, 105
  thalamic reticular nucleus, 111
  ventral anterior nucleus, 109
  ventral lateral nucleus, 109
  ventral posterolateral nucleus, 109
  ventral posteromedial nucleus, 109–110
Third ventricle, 191
Tic douloureux, 77
Tourette syndrome, 135
Transcalvarial herniation, 230
Transcortical sensory aphasia, 185
Transverse myelitis, 20
Transverse sinuses, 213
Traumatic spinal cord injury
  anterior cord syndrome, 18
  Brown-Séquard syndrome, 17

Traumatic spinal cord injury (*cont.*)
 central cord syndrome, 17–18
 complete transection, 17
 conus medullaris vs. cauda equina syndrome, 18
 posterior cord syndrome, 18
Trigeminal ganglion, 73
Trigeminal nerve, 41
 clinical relevance, 72–78
 functional classification, 72
 mandibular division, 75
 maxillary division, 74
 nuclear organization, 73
 ophthalmic division, 74
 overview, 72
Trigeminal neuralgia, 77
Trigeminothalamic tracts, 55
Trk receptor signaling pathways, 246–247
Trochlear nerve, 37
 clinical relevance, 71, 72
 course and distribution, 71
 functional classification, 70
 nuclear origin and unique anatomical features, 70
 superior oblique muscle, 71
Tuberculosis of the spine, 22
Tuberomammillary nucleus, 53

U

Uncal herniation, 230
Upward cerebellar herniation, 231

V

Vagus nerve, 49
Vascular disorders, 21
Vascular supply, 13, 14, 119–120
Vascular watersheds, 14
Venous drainage, 14, 184
Ventral amygdalofugal pathway, 114, 170
Ventral anterior nucleus, 109
Ventral lateral nucleus, 109
Ventral pallidum, 130
Ventral posterolateral nucleus, 109
Ventral posteromedial nucleus, 109–110
Ventral tegmental area (VTA), 50, 130, 131
Ventricular system
 anatomical components
  central canal, 192–193
  cerebral aqueduct, 192
  fourth ventricle, 192
  lateral ventricles, 190–191
  third ventricle, 191
 cerebrospinal fluid dynamics, 193–194
Ventriculoperitoneal shunt, 200
Ventromedial prefrontal cortex (VMPFC), 147, 155
Vertebrobasilar system, 206–208
Vestibulocerebellum, 86–87
Vestibulocochlear nerve, 42
Visual agnosias, 162
Visual field defects, 161–162
Visual field representation, 160
Visual processing, 161
Visual recognition disorders, 166

W

Waardenburg syndrome, 240
Walker-Warburg syndrome, 256
Wernicke encephalopathy, 120
Wernicke-Korsakoff syndrome, 120, 121
Wernicke's aphasia, 165, 166, 185
Wernicke's area, 149
White matter (myelinated axon tracts), 1

Z

Zona incerta, 119
Zygomatic nerve, 75

The manufacturer's authorised representative in the EU is Springer Nature Customer Service Centre GmbH, Europaplatz 3, 69115 Heidelberg, Germany. If you have any concerns regarding our products, please contact ProductSafety@springernature.com

Printed and bound by CPI Group (UK) Ltd, Croydon, CR0 4YY

07/07/2026

02160912-0001